CASTLE CONNOLLY MEDICAL LTD.

John K. Castle, Chairman
John L Connolly, Ed.D. President & CEO

www.castleconnolly.com

W9-CZV-946

Dear Friend,

The holiday season is upon us and as a way of sharing it's joy I have enclosed a copy of our newest Castle Connolly Guide, *America's Cosmetic Doctors and Dentists*.

Whether or not you are among the more than 10 million Americans who each year have a cosmetic treatment or surgery performed, or among the many millions more who are considering it, you will find this book of interest.

Not only does it describe all a patient needs to know about most major cosmetic procedures and treatments, but it contains listings of more than 6,000 physicians and dentists whose credentials we have reviewed to be certain they are properly trained to offer cosmetic care. The book is unique in another respect: the biographies of these cosmetic doctors and dentists are located on an Internet site that is made accessible by the CD-ROM enclosed in the back cover. You may also "link" from our site to the practice websites of many of the physicians and dentists listed.

We hope you will enjoy this gift from your colleagues at Castle Connolly Medical Ltd. and we wish you a wonderful holiday season and healthy and successful New Year.

Best Regards,

John J. Connolly, Ed.D.
President & CEO

the trusted source for healthcare choices

America's
Cosmetic
Doctors *and* Dentists

Consumer Guide

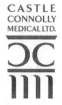

CASTLE
CONNOLLY
MEDICAL LTD.

A CASTLE CONNOLLY GUIDE

All Rights Reserved

Copyright © 2003, by Castle Connolly Medical Ltd.

Library of Congress Catalog Card Number 2003100262

This guide is designed to provide information of a general nature about elective care procedures. The information is provided with the understanding that Castle Connolly Medical Ltd. is not engaged in rendering any form of medical advice, professional services or recommendations. Any information contained herein should not be considered a substitute for medical advice provided by a qualified physician, surgeon, dentist and/or other appropriate health care professional to address your individual medical needs. Your particular facts and circumstances will determine the treatment that is most appropriate for you. Consult your own physician and/or other appropriate health care professional on specific medical questions, including matters requiring diagnosis, treatment, therapy or medical attention. The information contained in this report is delivered "as-is" without any form of warranty expressed or implied. Any use of the information contained within is solely at your own risk. Castle Connolly Medical Ltd. assumes no liability or responsibility for any claims, actions, or damages resulting from information provided in any article of advertisement contained herein. The contents of this guide including, but not limited to text, graphics and icons, are copyrighted property of Castle Connolly Medical Ltd. Reproduction, redistribution or modification in any form by any means of the information contained herein for any purpose is strictly prohibited. While all physicians and dentists listed on the attached CD ROM meet certain criteria established by Castle Connolly Medical Ltd., no guarantees can be made by Castle Connolly Medical Ltd. or its representatives regarding the expertise of the individual surgeons profiled. Reproduction in whole or part, or storage in any data retrieval system and reproduction therefrom, is strictly prohibited and violates federal copyright and trademark laws.

"The confidence of our readers in our editorial integrity is crucial to the success of the Castle Connolly Guides. Any use of the Castle Connolly name, or of any list or listing (or portion of either) from any Castle Connolly Guide, for advertising or for any commercial purpose, without prior written consent, is strictly prohibited and may result in legal action."

For more information, please contact Castle Connolly Medical Ltd., 42 West 24th St, New York, New York 10010, 212-367-8400 x10
E-mail: info@castleconnolly.com. Web site: http://www.castleconnolly.com

ISBN 1-883769-35-3 (paperback)
ISBN 1-883769-39-6 (hardcover)

Printed in the United States of America

America's
Cosmetic
Doctors and Dentists

Consumer Guide

**Text by: Wendy Lewis and
John J. Connolly Ed. D.**

A CASTLE CONNOLLY GUIDE

What Physician Leaders Say About
Americas Cosmetic Doctors and Dentists

"Reading this very informative book should help many people contemplating cosmetic surgery or related treatments to understand the variety of options available to them. It is a terrific first step in preparing for a meaningful interview with a qualified plastic surgery specialist, such as a member of the American Society for Aesthetic Plastic Surgery, and in achieving ultimate satisfaction from cosmetic surgery."

Robert W. Bernard, MD, White Plains, NY
President, American Society for Aesthetic Plastic Surgery

"Dentists with extensive experience in the expanding field of cosmetic dentistry use both science and artistry to help individuals create the smile they most desire. Experienced cosmetic dentists are up-to-date on the latest techniques and are the best resource for someone who is seeking a professional to redesign their smile. With the wide array of techniques that are now available, it's important that you consult with an experienced cosmetic dentist to discuss your treatment plan. This will ensure that you are advised on the most appropriate solutions to create your new smile."

Mike Malone, DDS, FAGD
President of the American Academy of Cosmetic Dentistry

"Prior to undergoing facial plastic surgery it is imperative to gain as much information about your surgery as possible. As an informed patient you will be able to work with the surgeon to get the best outcome. This guide will help provide the information necessary to become an informed patient."

Dean M. Toriumi, MD, Professor
Division of Facial Plastic and Reconstructive Surgery
Department of Otolaryngology-Head & Neck Surgery
University of Illinois at Chicago

About Castle Connolly Medical Ltd.

The trusted source for healthcare choices

Castle Connolly Medical Ltd. is the research and information company nationally recognized for *America's Top Doctors*, a user friendly guide that profiles nearly 4,700 top referral specialists throughout the United States, and for the Top Doctors series of regional guides to finding the best healthcare. Regional guides are currently available for the New York metro area, the Chicago metropolitan area and the state of Florida. Physicians are selected for inclusion based on extensive mail and phone surveys of thousands of phycisians each year asking them to nominate the best in their medical specialties. In addition, the credentials of those ultimately included are thoroughly reviewed by the Castle Connolly physician-led research team.

Our website at castleconnolly.com, americastopdoctors.com, and americascosmeticdoctors.com provides information and features on the best doctors and hospitals in these regions and other health related guidance for consumers. Castle Connolly also offers information on quality healthcare choices through its Internet partnerships and alliances with NewYorkMetro.com and others.

Castle Connolly has collaborative relationships for top doctors' feature articles with national magazines such as *Ladies Home Journal, Redbook* and *Town & Country*, and with leading regional magazines, such as *New York, Atlanta, Chicago, San Francisco, St. Louis, Miami Metro* and *Jacksonville*.

Table of Contents

About The Publishers

John K. Castle, the Chairman of Castle Connolly Medical Ltd., has spent much of the last two decades involved with healthcare institutions and issues. Mr. Castle served as Chairman of the Board of New York Medical College for eleven years, an institution at which he has continued on the Board for more than twenty years.

Mr. Castle has been extensively involved in other healthcare and voluntary activities as well. He served for five years as a public commissioner on the Joint Commission on Accreditation of Healthcare Organizations (JCAHO), the body which accredits most public and private hospitals throughout the United States. Mr. Castle has also served as a trustee of five different hospitals in the metropolitan New York region and is a director emeritus of the United Hospital Fund as well as a trustee of the Whitehead Institute.

In addition to his healthcare activities, Mr. Castle has served on many voluntary boards including the Corporation of the Massachusetts Institute of Technology, as well as numerous corporate boards of directors, including the Equitable Life Assurance Society of the United States. He is chairman of a leading merchant bank and has been chief executive of a major investment bank.

Mr. Castle holds a Bachelor of Science degree from MIT, an MBA with High Distinction from the Harvard Business School, where he was a Baker Scholar, and an honorary doctorate from New York Medical College.

John J. Connolly, Ed.D. is the President & CEO of Castle Connolly Medical Ltd., the nation's foremost expert on identifying top physicians. His experience in healthcare is extensive.

Dr. Connolly served as President of New York Medical College, the nation's second largest private medical college, for more than ten years. He is a Fellow of the New York Academy of Medicine, a Fellow of the New York Academy of Sciences, a Director of the New York Business Group on Health, a member of the President's Council of the United Hospital Fund, and a member of the Board of Advisors of Funding First a Lasker Foundation Initiative. Dr. Connolly has served as a trustee of two hospitals and as Chairman of the Board of one. He is extensively involved in healthcare and community activities and serves on a number of voluntary and corporate boards including the Board of the American Lyme Disease Foundation, of which he is a founder and past chairman, and the Board of Advisors of the Whitehead Institute for Biomedical Research. He is also the Chairman of AlphaGene Inc., a genomics research company in Woburn Massachusetts. He holds a Bachelor of Science degree from Worcester State College, a Master's degree from the University of Connecticut, and a Doctor of Education degree in College and University Administration from Teacher's College, Columbia University.

Dr. Connolly has appeared on or been interviewed by more than 100 television and radio stations nationwide including "Good Morning America" (ABC-TV), "20/20" (ABC-TV), "48 Hours" (CBS-TV), Fox Cable News (national), "Morning News" (CNN) and "Weekend Today in New York" (WNBC-TV), *The New York Times*, the *Chicago Tribune*, the *Daily News* (New York), the *Boston Herald* and other newspapers, as well as many national and regional magazines, have featured Castle Connolly Guides and/or Dr. Connolly in stories. Magazine coverage has included *Fortune, Town & Country, Money Magazine, New York Magazine, San Francisco Magazine, Chicago Magazine, Atlanta Magazine* and others.

Medical Advisory Board

We are pleased to have associated with Castle Connolly Medical Ltd. a distinguished group of medical leaders who offer invaluable advice and wisdom in our efforts to assist consumers in making the best healthcare choices. We thank each member of the Medical Advisory Board for their valuable contributions.

Charles Bechert, M.D.
The Sight Foundation
Fort Lauderdale, FL

Roger Bulger, M.D.
President and CEO
Association of Academic Health
Centers
Washington, DC

Harry J. Buncke, M.D.
Davies Medical Center
San Francisco, CA

Paul T. Calabresi, M.D.
Chairman Emeritus
Department of Medicine
Brown University
Rhode Island Hospital
Providence, RI

Joseph Cimino, M.D.
Professor and Chairman
Community and Preventive
Medicine
New York Medical College
Valhalla, NY

Jane Clark, M.D.
Ear, Nose, Throat, and Hearing
Center of Framingham
61 Lincoln St.
Framingham, MA

J. Richard Gaintner, M.D.
Chief Executive Officer (retired)
Shands Health Care
University of Florida
Gainesville, FL

Menard M. Gertler, M.D., D.Sc.
Clinical Professor of Medicine
Cornell University Medical School
New York, NY

Leo Hennikoff, M.D.
President and CEO (retired)
Rush Presbyterian-St.Luke's Medical
Center
Chicago, IL

Yutaka Kikkawa, M.D.
Professor and Chairman (Emeritus)
Department of Pathology
University of California, Irvine
College of Medicine
Irvine, CA

Nicholas F. LaRusso, M.D.
Chairman
Department of Medicine
Mayo Clinic
Rochester, MN

David Paige, M.D.
Professor
Bloomberg School of Public Health
Johns Hopkins University
Baltimore, MD

Ronald Pion, M.D.
Chairman and CEO
Medical Telecommunications
Associates
Los Angeles, CA

Richard L. Reece, M.D.
Editor
Physician Practice Options
Old Saybrook, CT

Leon G. Smith, M.D.
Chairman of Medicine
St. Michael's Medical Center
Newark, NJ

Helen Smits, M.D.
Former Deputy Director
Health Care Financing
Administration (HCFA)
New York, NY

Ralph Snyderman, M.D.
President and CEO
Duke University Health System
Durham, NC

Hippocratic Oath

I swear by Apollo the physician, and Asklepios, and health, and All-Heal and all the gods and goddesses, that, according to my ability and judgement, I will keep this Oath and this stipulation — to reckon him who taught me this Art equally dear to me as my parents, to share my substance with him, and relieve his necessities if required; to look upon his offspring in the same footing as my own brothers, and to teach them this Art, if they should wish to learn it, without fee or stipulation; and that by precept, lecture and every other mode of instruction, I will impart a knowledge of the Art to my own sons, and those of my teachers, and to disciples bound by a stipulation and oath according to the law of medicine, but to none others.

I will follow that system of regimen which, according to my ability and judgement, I consider for the benefit of my patients, and abstain from whatever is deleterious and mischievous. I will give no deadly medicine to anyone if asked nor suggest any such counsel; and in like manner I will not give to a woman a pessary to produce abortion. With purity and wholeness I will pass my life and practice my Art.

I will not cut persons labouring under the stone, but will leave this to be done by men who are practitioners of this work. Into whatever houses I enter, I will go into them for the benefit of the sick, and will abstain from every voluntary act of mischief and corruption; and, further, from the seduction of females or males, of freemen and slaves. Whatever, in connection with my professional practice, or not in connection with it, I see or hear, in the life of men, which ought not to be spoken of abroad, I will not divulge, as reckoning that all such should be kept secret. While I continue to keep this Oath unviolated, may it be granted to me to enjoy life and the practice of the art, respected by all men, in all times! But should I trespass and violate this Oath, may the reverse be my lot!

from Dorland's Illustrated Medical Dictionary. 27th ed. (Philadelphia) W.B. Saunders Co., 1988. Hippocratic Oath. [Hippocrates. Greek physician, 460-377 B.C.]

Foreword

Cosmetic Medicine Isn't "Cosmetic" Anymore

Dr. Steve Salvatore
Health Editor, Fox-5 News

You hold in your hands a guide to the many areas of medicine and health care that fall under the general rubric of Cosmetic Medicine. The word "cosmetic" has all sorts of connotations that we have inherited from a bygone era—a way of thinking that has become obsolete in ordinary life as it has in medical science. "Cosmetic" used to mean "superficial" and "insubstantial." A "cosmetic" adjustment meant something changed only on the surface, and only to make something look better than it really was—and that was true of a person's appearance no less than the front of a house or the decor in a living room. Not so very long ago, people going to a plastic surgeon for facial surgery or to a dermatologist for skin treatments would be considered vain, and such practices would be considered elective at best, and unnecessary at worst.

But our thinking has changed radically in the past decade. We now know that the medical specialists who work in the various fields of cosmetic medicine perform vital services, often vastly improving their patients' quality of life. This work ranges from the reconstructive procedures that are applied to accident and burn victims and to children born with deformities, to people who are seeking to improve their image—to themselves, to their loved ones and to their friends and colleagues. And as the population gets older, working and actively living to more advanced years, it is only natural to want to maintain the countenance our friends know, love and respect. This will require some serious maintenance on the part of patients, but in our competitive society, we will likely need help from some of the specialties cataloged here.

Many of the techniques and procedures developed by cosmetic medicine and dentistry were first applied to patients who needed them to lead normal lives. Now we are able to avail ourselves of these techniques and advances to maintain a vigorous and healthful appearance, to maintain an energetic and youthfully exuberant attitude and self-image, and to maintain our attractiveness to our spouse, our children, and to those who know us. This book will prove invaluable in attaining those goals—and there is nothing cosmetic about that.

section I

THE BEST CHOICES FOR YOU

A cosmetic treatment is not something you rush into lightly. It is a serious undertaking and can be expensive. It should be approached thoughtfully and with care. The most important issue to be addressed is the selection of a physician or dentist. That decision alone will be *the* major determinant of the success of your treatment. But there are other issues to consider as well. How do you find that "right" doctor or dentist? What kind of anesthesia will you need for your treatment? What will it cost? How will you pay for it? How can you better prepare to improve the probability of success in your treatment?

All of these are important issues to address even before you undertake a cosmetic treatment. Your major focus, however, will be on selecting the right doctor or dentist. Your personal feelings will be important in that choice, but there are other criteria, more objective ones perhaps, that are also critically important. Choosing a doctor may be almost as important as choosing a spouse. You shouldn't make either choice based on emotion alone.

This section of *America's Cosmetic Doctors and Dentists* will assist you in making the selection of a doctor or dentist wisely.

In addition, once you have decided on cosmetic treatments and selected a physician or dentist there is still some preparation called for on your part. You need to discuss where your treatment will take place and what anesthesia, if any, will be required. All of these issues, and more, will be dealt with in this introductory section.

chapter 1

"The largely objective character of beauty is further indicated by the fact that to a considerable extent beauty is the expression of health. A well and harmoniously developed body, tense muscles, an elastic and finely toned skin, bright eyes, grace and animation of carriage – all these things which are essential to beauty are the conditions of health."

Havelock Ellis

NOT EVERY DOCTOR IS THE RIGHT ONE

This book has been written, researched and compiled for the millions of whom seek cosmetic medical and dental care each year. There are more than eight million cosmetic procedures performed each year on 6.6 million Americans. It is very likely there are additional millions contemplating some kind of cosmetic treatment and this book is for them as well.

Cosmetic, or aesthetic care, like all medical and dental care, is extremely important to patients. In fact, to many people it can be the most important kind of care because it affects the image they present to others as well as their self image. In most cases, patients seek cosmetic care voluntarily and they pay for it from their own pockets. They are making an important investment – in themselves, their appearance and their future.

Why does Castle Connolly believe this book is necessary and will be invaluable to people considering cosmetic treatment?

You need only to look at newspaper and magazine headlines, listen to the radio or watch television news to fully appreciate the need for this guide. The media are all too frequently reporting on disasters as a result of cosmetic surgery. The stories of patients who are simply unhappy with their results never make the media, but we probably all know someone personally who falls into that group. Does this mean we should not consider cosmetic treatment? No, but it does mean we need to be scrupulously careful in choosing the right professional to do it because, unfortunately, there are people with little or no medical training who attempt to perform cosmetic procedures – often with devastating results.

There are also physicians and dentists who, although licensed, are not properly trained in cosmetic procedures and techniques, but are offering them. This is not a simple issue. Physicians are licensed to practice medicine by individual states, not by the federal government. In some states an individual can be licensed to practice medicine after graduating from medical school, completing just one year of a residency program and passing a state licensing exam. In other words, this doctor does not even have to complete an approved residency program, which is a minimum of three years.

> *There is no legal requirement in any state that requires that a physician have specific training in a specialty before practicing it!*

Furthermore, the doctor can go out and practice any medical specialty he or she chooses. That means they can call themselves cardiologists, pediatricians, psychiatrists, or cosmetic surgeons. There is no legal requirement in any state that requires that a physician have specific training in a specialty before practicing it. The practice of medicine is not restricted. Once someone is licensed as a physician or dentist, it is solely their professional judgment and ethics that control what they do to their patients, at least in their own office or clinic.

Many people are shocked when they hear this. They naturally assume that the government or the medical profession is protecting them by officially monitoring the situation.

Fortunately, there is a strong degree of professionalism and ethics among the overwhelming majority of physicians and dentists and they perform procedures and provide care only in areas for which they are appropriately trained. In addition, hospitals provide supervision of the care offered by physicians and dentists within their walls, reviewing credentials and approving the procedures a physician or dentist may perform – but only within the hospital. However, the majority of cosmetic procedures are offered outside of a hospital, so it is up to the physician or dentist to exercise appropriate professional judgment and it is up to the consumer to be certain the physician or dentist is appropriately trained.

It was with this goal, helping consumers be certain their physicians and dentists are appropriately trained and have the potential of providing the best care possible, that Castle Connolly created this guide.

In this guide we have gone further than simply outlining the process you should follow in order to identify a qualified physician or dentist for cosmetic care. We have done much of the work for you. Our physician-directed research team has screened the physicians and dentists included in our database to assure that they have been properly trained in their specialties. For the most part, this means those listed in our database are board certified, have not been disciplined by any state medical board, and have been trained appropriately for the procedures and techniques that are listed in this Guide. Nonetheless, our screening does not absolve the responsible patient from investigating the credentials of any physician or dentist they are considering. Ultimately, you have to choose a physician or dentist with whom you feel comfortable and trust. This guide will assist you in that process, but the ultimate choice will be yours.

We also took a somewhat unique approach in listing the biographies of the physicians and dentists. Instead of printing their professional bios, as we have with other Castle Connolly Guides, this registry will be accessible via an internet connection, utilizing software on the CD enclosed within this book. This allows us to continually update and enhance the registry.

Not only does this approach reduce the size and bulk of the book, but it means that you can do searches for physicians and dentists that meet your personal criteria by using your computer. For example, you could enter a city, (Los Angeles), a specialty (plastic surgery), and a procedure (face-lift) and our database would produce a list of physicians meeting those criteria.

Having links to the physician and dentist biographies offers our readers another major advantage. Many of the physicians and dentists have paid for an enhanced listing to establish a link from their biography in our database to their own website. (Important note: there is no fee to physicians or dentists to be screened and included in this guide. The charge is for the link to their website only.) These links will make it possible for you to learn more about the physician's or dentist's practice by linking to their practice website. Many physicians and dentists have extensive websites with before-and-after photos and a great deal of information about procedures, fees, scheduling and more. Visiting these websites can be a valuable learning experience and will assist you in knowing more about any doctor or dentist you may consider. In addition, by visiting a number of these websites you can learn about the different professional approaches in the field and better understand the many nuances underlying cosmetic treatment.

*"Even beauties can be unattractive. If you catch a beauty in the wrong light
at the right time, forget it. I believe in low lights and trick mirrors. I believe
in plastic surgery."*

-Andy Warhol

HOW WE IDENTIFIED THE DOCTORS AND DENTISTS

Castle Connolly Medical Ltd. is best known for its "Top Doctors" guides. In
these guides, published regionally in New York, Chicago and Florida, and
nationally as *America's Top Doctors*, physicians are selected based upon
extensive mail and phone surveys of physicians, medical school deans,
hospital chiefs of services, VPs for Medical Affairs, residency programs
directors and, in some cases, nurses. This extensive nomination process is
designed to identify those who are among the best in their respective specialties. After extensive mail surveys, the Castle Connolly physician-directed research team conducts thousands of phone interviews, validating and
reinforcing the information gathered from the mail surveys, and identifying
additional candidates for inclusion. Finally, after the thousands of physicians nominated are narrowed down to a select few, the research staff
checks on the disciplinary record of each physician.

A very important point: doctors and dentists do not and cannot pay to
be included in any of our guides, including this one.

In creating the listing and database for *America's Cosmetic Doctors and
Dentists*, Castle Connolly modified its selection method. Since so much of
cosmetic medical and dental practice does not take place in a hospital, a
physician or dentist does not work as closely with his/her colleagues as
they may in a typical acute care hospital setting. As a result, we did not
undertake our standard survey process.

Identifying all of the nation's physicians and dentists who are engaged
in cosmetic practice is not an easy task. In the United States there are

approximately 640,000 physicians and 150,000 dentists. Only a small percentage of these offer cosmetic care and an even smaller number are fully qualified to deliver cosmetic care.

To begin the identification process, we mailed letters to more than 30,000 board certified physicians in the following specialties: Plastic Surgery, Dermatology, Ophthalmology, and Otolaryngology (Head and Neck Surgery), as well as to dentists. In addition, we sent mailings to physicians who subscribe to *Cosmetic Surgery Times*, a professional journal in the field. We assumed that most of the subscribers were actively engaged in cosmetic practice. We also followed up our mailings with phone calls.

Since cosmetic treatment is something one can observe visually, many physicians and dentist have websites so that potential patients can see evidence of the quality of their work.

To identify dentists who offered cosmetic/aethestic care we mailed to the members of the American Academy of Cosmetic Dentistry. In addition, we followed up this group of dentists with phone calls.

Lastly, we searched the Internet to identify both qualified physicians and dentists engaged in cosmetic practice. Since cosmetic treatment is something one can observe visually, many physicians and dentists have websites so that potential patients can see evidence of the quality of their work. We contacted as many of the physicians and dentists in this category as we could identify. It is possible that we have missed some who meet these criteria. If so, we invite them to contact us so we may review their credentials and, if appropriate, include them in our database. There may be others who wish to add a "link" to their bios, which can be accomplished at any time.

After gathering the professional biographical information on each physician and dentist, our physician-directed research team reviewed their credentials, including medical school, residency, fellowships, hospital appointments and special expertise. The research team often called and requested more information or clarification on their training and, finally, before deciding to include a physician or dentist, we checked with the states to be certain they had not been disciplined by a state medical board or other licensing agency. This latter step is a good one for any prospective patient to undertake any time they are considering a new physician or dentist. To assist you in that process we have included a list of the agencies responsible for maintaining such data and the phone number, website (if the information is available online), and physical address. (Appendix A)

Our approach to identifying and screening physicians and dentists for this guide is to assume that physicians whose specialties are Plastic Surgery, Dermatology, Otolaryngology, Ophthalmology and dentists whose specialty is Oral Maxillofacial Surgery (with a medical degree) could have been trained in cosmetic procedures during their residency, fellowships or, at times, later in Continuing Medical Education (CME) programs. The notion that these physicians could have been trained does not mean they were trained or have incorporated cosmetics into their practices. Furthermore, the specific cosmetic techniques each specialty is trained to perform differs.

The area of a physician's "Special Expertise", that is the specific procedures they claim expertise in, is a complex one. It is not enough, in our opinion, for a physician to be licensed, or even board certified, to perform all cosmetic procedures. They must have had specific training in the treatments and procedures being offered. In determining this, we followed the training requirements spelled out by the governing boards of each specialty.

For example, according to the American Academy of Dermatology, dermatologists may be trained in "small volume liposuction", so we will list that procedure in the biographies of many dermatologists in our database. However, according to their own medical governing board, dermatologists are not trained in "large volume liposuction", so we would not permit a dermatologist who requested it to list procedures requiring that technique.

Similarly, while many ophthalmologists are trained to do eyelid surgery, few are trained to do full face-lifts, so we would not list that procedure as the special expertise of an ophthalmologist.

Yet, even those trained to do a procedure during a residency or fellowship, or who learned it later, may not choose to incorporate cosmetic procedures in their practice. Many dermatologists may do some superficial chemical peels but do not consider cosmetics part of their practice. Many ophthalmologists do not perform aesthetic surgery of the eyelids, and many plastic surgeons perform only burn and reconstructive surgery, and not cosmetic work.

Our efforts were focused on identifying physicians and dentists who are, first, actively engaged in cosmetic/aesthetic practice and, second, properly trained.

Our efforts were focused on identifying physicians and dentists who are, first, actively engaged in cosmetic/aesthetic practice and, second, properly trained. Our research led us to identify and include more than 6,300 physicians and dentists who meet both criteria.

While we cannot guarantee to you that a physician or dentist is outstanding, we can assure you that they are appropriately trained for cosmetic care and have not experienced serious disciplinary issues in the past. The final choice will be yours and will depend on your individual preferences. Hopefully, the guidance offered in this text will assist you in that process.

"Basically, the difference between good surgery and bad is the difference between looking younger and better or like something out of a wax museum."

E!ONLINE
Sally Ogle Davis and Ivor Davis

CHOOSING THE RIGHT DOCTOR OR DENTIST FOR COSMETIC CARE

In the realm of cosmetic surgery and treatments, there is rarely only one best doctor or dentist for any procedure. There are usually many who can execute an excellent result. Ultimately, the decision of selecting a physician or dentist is yours and yours alone. No one can really make the choice for you, nor should they. However, determining who is best for you is no small feat. You can't just go up to a woman in a store and ask, "Who did your face?", although many have done exactly that.

If you have been considering having some cosmetic work done, you probably have been collecting names of doctors from friends, physicians and others, along with clippings from magazines and newspapers; each source has its own favorites. Although recommendations from friends and acquaintances can be helpful, it isn't fair to judge a doctor or dentist on the basis of one isolated recommendation or condemnation either.

The main concern for anyone considering surgery should be, "Who is the best doctor for ME?"

The most important credential a doctor or dentist has is his or her professional reputation. The "best" doctor for your sister-in-law may not be the right one for you for a variety of reasons. The main concern of anyone considering surgery should be, "Who is the best doctor for ME?"

There are also credentials of excellence that you have to make certain are in place before selecting a doctor. The following section describes those credentials and how you can assess them.

The physicians and dentists who are listed in this guide include dentists, oral maxillofacial surgeons (some of whom have both medical and dental degrees), and physicians in the following specialties: Plastic Surgery; Dermatology; Ophthalmology; and Otolaryngology (head and neck surgery). We have included these specialties because they are the only medical specialties in which physicians receive specific cosmetic training. We also have included a small number of general surgeons who treat varicose veins, a procedure that may be viewed as cosmetic for some patients.

There are physicians in other medical specialties who perform cosmetic surgery and treatments that we have not included in this guide. However, we would caution consumers about seeking cosmetic care from physicians who are not trained in the specialties described because, although there may be some who have returned to a fellowship or another extensive training program in order to be trained appropriately for cosmetic care, that is generally not the case. In fact, some physicians are adding cosmetic treatments to their practices simply because it generates additional revenue, unencumbered by the bureaucracy of insurance companies and hospitals.

Cosmetic Treatment Offered By Non-Physicians

Cosmetic treatment is a growing business. Unfortunately, as in any growth industry, there are many people who attempt to take advantage of the opportunities presented and this is as true in the cosmetic field as in any other field. While some of these people may be well-trained in their profession, they are simply not qualified to provide cosmetic medical or dental services. This group includes people who have no medical training at all, or others with minimal medical training, or perhaps training in a health profession other than medicine or dentistry. They look towards cosmetic treatment purely as a money-making opportunity.

In addition, patients should be wary of physicians who may be trained in a specialty that does not include cosmetic care but who are offering these services because of the financial returns possible. Cosmetic procedures, either medical or dental, are a serious issue and many have the potential for death or disfigurement if not performed properly. Some of these procedures may seem simple, such as botulinum toxin treatments, but, occasionally, even the seemingly simplest procedures can lead to serious complications. If all goes well it may seem fine to go to someone other than an appropriately trained physician for certain minimally invasive treatments. However, if things don't go well, the talents of a skilled and well-trained physician or dentist may become mandatory.

chapter 4

"Americans spend more each year on beauty than they do on education. Such spending is not mere vanity. Being pretty-or just not ugly-confers an enormous genetic and social advantage"

The Beauty Business: Pots of Promise.
The Economist May 24, 2003

IDENTIFYING YOUR OWN BEST DOCTOR OR DENTIST

When searching for a doctor or dentist, whether it is for cosmetic treatment or any type of health need, we should always take the utmost care. Selecting a doctor or dentist is among the most important choices we make. We are choosing professionals to trust not only with our looks and health, but also our lives.

Yet, all too often we choose a doctor or dentist in a very casual fashion. Some of us will spend more time deciding what car to buy, what movie to attend, or even at which restaurant to dine, than we will in selecting a doctor or dentist. And there are no test drives when it comes to medical treatment. We may ask a friend, or simply look-up a name in a phone book or our health plan directory. The location of the doctor's office may be the primary piece of information we consider.

The fact you are using this guide demonstrates you intend to be more careful and more selective and that's a great start. But what should you look for in choosing a doctor or dentist for cosmetic care?

The first criteria, one we have touched upon previously, is the doctor's basic qualifications. Most importantly, is the doctor board certified in one of the specialties that are the focus of this guide: Plastic Surgery, Dermatology, Ophthalmology, Otolaryngology or Oral Maxillofacial Surgery? Has the dentist had training in the cosmetic procedures you are considering and is he or she accredited by the American Academy of Cosmetic Dentistry?

As you read earlier, board certification assures you, the patient, that the doctor has graduated from an accredited medical school and, after medical school, completed an approved residency program of at least three years, and passed a certifying exam. Board certification does not guarantee a great doctor,

Board certification does not guarantee a great doctor, but it at least assures you the physician has been appropriately trained for that specialty.

but it at least assures you the physician has been appropriately trained for that specialty. (To check on a doctor's board certification call the ABMS, American Board of Medical Specialties, at 866-ASK-ABMS or visit their website at www.ABMS.org. For DOs, Doctors of Osteopathic Medicine, you may check their credentials by calling the American Osteopathic Association at 800-621-1773.)

What is a Medical Specialist?

This guide deals with a specific group of medical specialists, all of whom are trained to provide some cosmetic care. The dental profession also has specialties and specific cosmetic training that will be described later in this chapter.

This team "specialist" is used liberally by both laypeople and medical professionals and it is frequently used incorrectly. One of the reasons for this is that there is no restriction, legal or otherwise, against its improper use. Technically, a medical specialist is a physician who has completed an approved residency of at least three years duration and passed an exam in a specialty approved by the American Board of Medical Specialists (ABMS). The 24 member boards of the ABMS issue general certification in 25 specialties and 90 subspecialties. When a physician has completed an approved residency program, all of which are at least three years in length and in some specialties longer, and sits for, and passes, an extensive board exam, he or she is considered "board-certified" and is called a "fellow" of that specialty. The ABMS is the governing body for, and approves, the specialty boards for MDs.

For Doctors of Osteopathic Medicine (DO), the approval body is the American Osteopathic Association (AOA). Under the AOA, there are 30 specialties and 73 subspecialties. Three of the Osteopathic specialties have cosmetic care as part of their training in residency and/or fellowship programs. They are Plastic Surgery, Dermatology, and Otolaryngology and Ophthalmology. (The latter two are combined in Osteopathic Medicine.)

A dental/medical specialty, Oral Maxillofacial Surgery, also has cosmetic surgery elements in its training program.

In addition to the medical boards recognized by the ABMS, there is another credential that should be taken seriously by consumers. That certification, by the American Board of Facial, Plastic and Reconstructive Surgery, is a meaningful credential that demands completion of a year-long fellowship training program, written and oral exams, peer review of at least 100 facial/plastic surgeries and prior certification in either Plastic Surgery or Otolayrngology. This board certification is sought primarily by otolayrngologists interested in cosmetic practice.

Although physicians who are board certified in these specialties are trained and qualified to do cosmetic procedures, they are not all equally qualified to perform the same procedures. For example, you would not choose an ophthalmologist for a breast enhancement. While that may be an obvious example, the selection of the appropriate specialists for some other procedures is less clear.

It is perfectly legal for a physicians to label themselves as any kind of specialist they choose and to perform treatments and procedures related to that specialty, however untrained they may be. Furthermore, there are some 130 groups that call themselves "specialties" that are not recognized by the ABMS. The ABMS calls these groups "self-designated medical specialties" and they are listed in Appendix B.

Some of these self-designated medical specialties have standards for membership, others are simply groups of physicians interested in an area of practice with no membership standards other than annual dues. A number of these groups are attempting to bring standards to these areas of medical practice, often with the goal of ultimately being recognized by the ABMS. Groups interested in cosmetic practices are; Aesthetic Plastic Surgery, Cosmetic Plastic Surgery, Cosmetic Surgery, Facial Cosmetic Surgery, Facial

The following are descriptions of the four ABMS recognized medical specialties in which physicians who are board certified have been trained to perform cosmetic procedures.

DERMATOLOGY

A dermatologist is trained to diagnose and treat pediatric and adult patients with benign and malignant disorders of the skin, mouth, external genitalia, hair and nails, as well as a number of sexually transmitted diseases. They also have expertise in the management of cosmetic disorders of the skin such as hair loss and scars and the skin changes associated with aging. The residency program is four years.

OPHTHALMOLOGY

An ophthalmologist has the knowledge and professional skills needed to provide comprehensive eye and vision care. Ophthalmologists are medically trained to diagnose, monitor and medically or surgically treat ocular and visual disorders. This includes problems affecting the eye and its component structures, the eyelids, the orbit and the visual pathways. The residency program is two years. Some ophthalmologists also perform plastic and reconstructive surgical procedures. They are typically known as Oculoplastic Surgeons. The fellowship training program is two years.

OTOLARYNGOLOGY

An otolaryngologist (head and neck surgeon) provides comprehensive medical and surgical care for patients with diseases and disorders that affect the ears, nose, throat, the respiratory and upper alimentary systems and related structures of the head and neck. Head and neck oncology, facial plastic and reconstructive surgery and the treatment of disorders of hearing and voice are fundamental areas of expertise. The residency training program is five years.

PLASTIC SURGERY

A plastic surgeon deals with the repair, reconstruction or replacement of physical defects of form or function involving the skin, muscoskeletal system, craniomaxillofacial structures, hand, extremities, breast and trunk and external genitalia. He/she uses aesthetic surgical principles not only to improve undesirable qualities of normal structures (commonly called "cosmetic surgery"), but in all reconstructive procedures as well. The residency training program is five years.

Plastic and Reconstructive Surgery, International Cosmetic Plastic Facial Reconstructive Surgery, Laser Surgery, and Plastic Esthetic Surgery.

While none of these groups is recognized by the ABMS, membership of a physician at least demonstrates an interest in cosmetic care. However, to stress again, it is board certification in Plastic Surgery, Dermotology, Otolarygology, Ophthalmology, or Oral Maxillofacial Surgery that is the most meaningful credential, but even that should be enhanced by additional training in specific cosmetic techniques and procedures.

"You're never too young to be younger."

Zsa Zsa Gabor, Actress

AREAS OF CONTROVERSY

After you have selected a physician who is board certified in an appropriate specialty you may feel your job of finding a good physician is over. However, that is just the beginning. There are some procedures where there is significant debate about the training of physicians required to perform them. At first glance it may seem obvious; ophthalmologists are trained to do cosmetic work around the eyes; otolaryngologists do surgery of the head and neck; dermatologists perform treatments on the skin and some dermatologists, dermatologic surgeons,

> *. . . we wish to make clear the position of the authors regarding having cosmetic procedures and treatments performed by physicians who are not board certified in these specialties: DO NOT!*

perform surgery of the skin, such as removing moles, skin cancer repairs and laser surgery; plastic surgeons are trained to do plastic and reconstructive surgery of the entire body.

Most physicians in these specialties restrict themselves to the generally accepted procedures and treatments deemed appropriate for their specialty. However, there are some gray areas and others where some physicians are aggressively pushing the boundaries of what, historically, has been practiced in their specialties.

First, we wish to make clear the position of the authors regarding having cosmetic procedures and treatments performed by physicians who are not board certified in these specialties: DO NOT! We do not believe it is worth the risk, however simple the procedure may seem. For example, some women visiting their primary care physician have seen signs in the office, or buttons worn by staff, posing the question, "Ask me about BOTOX®." While BOTOX® injections seemingly may be simple to perform, and some primary care physicians may have taken brief training programs, BOTOX® treatment should be part of a cosmetic care plan that may be best integrated with other kinds of cosmetic care. Therefore, it is in the best interests of the patient to have that care delivered by someone trained in cosmetic care generally and not simply a single procedure.

While it is legal for any licensed physician to perform cosmetic procedures, it is not in the patient's best interests and that is what is paramount.

Liposuction: Although liposuction was developed and popularized by an obstetrician/gynecologist in France, Dr. Yves-Gerard Illouz, it is a procedure performed primarily by plastic surgeons. In recent years a growing number of dermatologists, as well as some general surgeons, have been doing liposuction. Consumers should be careful about having liposuction performed by physicians not in these specialties and, furthermore, they have to look carefully into the training and experience of any physician they are considering for this procedure.

The primary concern regarding liposuction is the training of a physician to not only handle the cosmetic outcomes involved, but also to manage the issues of fluid shifts that occur during the surgical procedure. Physicians trained as surgeons have this experience as part of their residency training, whereas other physicians may not.

The other issue related to liposuction is large volume liposuction. Large volume liposuction is defined as the removal of approximately 5,000 cc's of fat or more, which is roughly equivalent to one and a quarter gallons. Most medical guidelines recommend that anytime that level of fat removal is approached it should be done in an approved surgical facility or an acute care hospital. If more than that is to be removed, it is advisable that it be performed in more than one stage.

In some states, legislation has been passed requiring that physicians , in order to perform liposuction in any setting, should have privileges to perform it in a hospital. This may be a growing movement as a way to protect patients. In part, this movement is attributable to the high death rate for liposuction as compared to other types of surgeries. In the right hands, liposuction can be a wonderful experience with rewarding results. In the wrong hands, it can be a life-threatening procedure for the patient.

In any case, a patient should have satisfying answers to the following two questions:

- Is the physician trained to do the procedure? Is the physician not just board certified, but has he or she been specifically trained in liposuction? Where? For how long? Was the training approved for Continuing Medical Education credit?

- Is the facility an accredited one? This is especially critical if the volume of fat to be removed approaches 4,000 - 5,000 cc's. An accredited surgical facility is prepared and equipped to deal with all emergencies. A doctor's office or operating suite may not be. (For resources on facility accreditation, see Appendix C.)

Facial Cosmetic Surgery: Cosmetic surgery of the face is another area consumers should approach with special care. Obviously, if you are going to invest in some kind of facial cosmetic treatment, be it surgical or dermatological, you want the very best outcome. Therefore, patients have to be cautious in their selection of a physician.

Four ABMS approved medical specialties and one dental/medical specialty include training in aspects of facial cosmetic surgery – of different types, however:

Ophthalmologists receive some training in occuplastic surgery. Dermatologists receive training in removing minor skin lesions and those trained in Procedural Dermatology, a new sub-specialty, receive training in dermatologic surgery, which includes small volume liposuction and hair transplants. Otolaryngologists receive training in cosmetic as well as reconstructive surgery of the head and neck, as do oral maxillofacial surgeons, especially those in MD/DDS programs. Of course, plastic and reconstructive surgeons are trained to perform plastic surgery on the entire body.

As a result, all of these doctors may claim that they are trained to do cosmetic surgery of the face.

Generally, ophthalmologists will work only on the eyes. Dermatologists will perform treatment only on the skin. If a physician in these specialties is doing more, their credentials and training

Any physician seriously committed to cosmetic practice will make the investment necessary to create an album of before and after photos.

for other procedures needs to be carefully scrutinized and should include extensive – months or years – of training. Even though all plastic surgeons are trained to do facial cosmetic surgery, a patient should ask the surgeon about their special training in specific procedures.

The same is true for otolaryngolgists. While they are all trained to do some cosmetic surgery of the face, a patient is well-advised to seek out those certified by the American Board of Facial, Plastic and Reconstructive Surgery.

Oral maxillofacial surgeons also are trained to do cosmetic surgery of the face, but since there is no ABMS recognized sub-certification available to them a patient needs to discuss in depth the training and experience of the surgeon.

The question for the potential patient, whether in selecting a plastic surgeon, dermatologist, ophthalmologist, otolaryngologist or oral maxillofacial surgeon, all of whom may claim to have been trained in cosmetic surgery of the face, are:

- Where were you trained?

- How long was the training period?

- How were you trained in this particular procedure?

- How many of this procedure have you performed?

- What has been your success rate?

It is appropriate to ask for evidence of a physician's education, training and experience. Well trained physicians are proud of their credentials and will often tell you about their training even before you ask them. The fancy documents framed on the office walls of most physicians and dentists are not there simply for decoration. You can tell you a lot about a doctor by what you find on their walls. They should tell you where he or she went to medical school, did their residency, their fellowships, board certification, special training in cosmetics, and memberships in medical societies and organizations. Most physicians in the cosmetic specialties also have a website and a practice brochure that may describe all of their training. Furthermore, always ask for before and after photographs. Any physician seriously committed to cosmetic practice will make the investment necessary to create an album of before and after photos.

All of this may seem daunting, but it is not. There is a system of specialties in place that has been created by medical and dental professionals who are as concerned about the safety and welfare of patients as they are about the art and science of their work. Using these specialties, and related board certification, as a guide, will help you identify a well trained physician or dentist. However, you still need to carefully explore that professional's experience, results and personality in order to choose the one that is right for you.

We have explained the system and its many nuances. If you follow it, and behave as an empowered and assertive consumer, you will enhance your chances of finding qualified and well-trained physicians and dentists and avoid making a mistake you may come to regret later.

chapter 6

"Talent counts thirty percent; appearance counts seventy."
Chinese proverb

CONSIDERING COSMETIC DENTISTRY

Finding the right cosmetic dentist can be more challenging because dentistry does not have an approved specialty for cosmetics. However, dentistry does have eight specialty areas. They are:

Endodontist: This specialist is concerned with the prevention, diagnosis and treatment of disorders of dental pulp that lies within the tooth. One of the most common procedures these dentists perform is a root canal.

Oral and Maxillofacial Surgeon: This specialist provides a broad range of diagnostic and treatment services for diseases, injuries and defects in the head, neck, face, jaw and associated structures. This specialty requires a minimum of four additional years of training once dental school is completed. Many oral maxillofacial surgeons have a MD degree as well as a DDS.

Oral Pathologist: This specialist is concerned with study and research into diseases of the mouth. Oral pathologists are often called to provide diagnostic and consultation services to general dentists.

Orthodontist: This specialist is concerned with problems related to crooked and missing teeth. These dentists work to help establish both normal dental function and improved personal appearance.

Pediatric Dentist: This specialist is concerned with treating children's dental needs from birth through adolescence.

Periodontist: This specialist is concerned with the diagnosis and treatment of the gums and the bone supporting the teeth. This specialty requires three additional years of training beyond basic dental school.

Prosthodontist: This specialist replaces missing natural teeth with fixed or removable structures such as dentures, bridges, or implants. This specialty requires three additional years of training beyond dental school.

> *The American Academy of Cosmetic Dentistry standards for accreditation include a written examination, submission of clinical case reports, and an oral examination.*

Public Health Dentist: This specialist is concerned with preventing and controlling dental disease in large population groups. These dentists work with public health officials to promote good dental care through organized community efforts.

Two of these specialties, Orthodontics and Prosthedonics, could be considered cosmetic because the results of their care include enhanced appearance as well as improved dental health. When undertaking sophisticated cosmetic dentistry, such as crowns and veneers, or anytime tooth color, matching, or a "re-do" of a full smile is desired, it is best to seek out a dentist accredited by the American Academy of Cosmetic Dentistry (AACD). The American Academy of Cosmetic Dentistry standards for accreditation include a written examination, submission of clinical case reports, and an oral examination. The AACD accredits both dentists and technicians. To maintain certification a dentist or technician must attend AACD scientific session on a regular basis.

In some areas it may not be possible to find an AACD accredited dentist, or a dentist may have had appropriate training but chose not to pursue AACD accreditation. In such cases you need to verify their training and experience. In doing so, you should ask the following questions:

- How many times have you performed this procedure?

- Where were you trained to perform the procedure? By Whom?

- How many have you performed before?

- Do you have photographs of your work?

Before and after photographs may seem somewhat superficial, but any dentist sincerely interested in developing a cosmetic practice will devote the time and money to compile them.

chapter 7

The top five surgical cosmetic procedures in 2002 were nose reshaping (354,327), liposuction (282,876), breast enlargement (236,888), eyelid surgery (230,672) and face lifts (117,831).

The American Society of Plastic Surgeons, ©2003

GETTING THE MOST FROM THE CONSULTATION

Before scheduling a consultation with a physician or dentist, request brochures describing the doctor's practice and develop a list of questions in order to discuss what is involved with a specific procedure. Force yourself to become Internet savvy or enlist the services of someone who can help you. Most doctors and dentists who have cosmetic practices will have their own website or a personal web page connected to their professional organization. (See appendix C for listings of professional organizations). Visit their websites, request their bio, CV, or practice brochure and materials about the procedures you are investigating. Get to know as much as you can about the doctor or dentist before you make the appointment to save your valuable time and money. Other factors to consider are fees, availability, and your impression of how helpful and organized the staff is. Find out in advance about the range of fees so you can be prepared to stay within your budget. If you have a specific date in mind, some physicians are booked way in advance, but there is sometimes a waiting list for cancellations if you are willing to be flexible. Once your initial list is narrowed down, start scheduling your consultation visits.

It is reasonable to expect a physician or dentist to charge a fee for his or her time. Most reputable doctors and dentists will charge a consultation fee of from $75 up to as much as $350. The consultation visit can run fifteen minutes to a full hour in some cases. Find out beforehand if you will be charged an additional fee for a second consultation. Most doctors charge only the one consultation fee, even if you come back two or three times before your procedure. However, consultation fees can add up if you will be seeing several doctors. If you do your homework ahead of time,

27

you may be able to rule out some of the doctors on your list based on what you find out even before you make your appointment.

Key Questions to Ask

It is common practice in cosmetic surgery for a doctor to hand you a mirror at the beginning of the consultation and ask you to show him or her what is bothering you, "What can I do for you?" It is your responsibility to communicate your goals to the doctor or dentist. You are not expected to know exactly what you need on your own, but you should be able to explain as specifically as possible what you don't like about your face, body or smile, what looks different or not as good as it used to, and what you want to change or improve. Don't arrive at your consultation appointment with a blank slate. Most practitioners hate to be asked the ubiquitous question, "What would you do to me?" Prepare a list of questions to bring with you to your consultation visit so you don't forget anything important to ask, and do take notes. You may forget most of what he or she tells you during the initial visit and writing it all down will come in handy later. Save the questions about fees, payment and scheduling for the doctor's secretary. If you get nervous during the consultation you can easily forget something that may be important to ask. You need to know the basics of the procedure and how they apply directly to you specifically. Understanding the limitations of the procedure is also crucial. Skin type, degree of skin elasticity, individual healing, bone structure, general health, dental health, previous surgery to the area, and many other factors will determine to some extent the quality of the result you can expect.

> *Prepare a list of questions to bring with you to your consultation visit so you don't forget anything important to ask, and do take notes.*

The Need to Know

- Find out how many incisions you will have and where they will be placed.
- Ask what kind of anesthesia will be given and who will be administering it.
- Inquire about the facility where the surgery will be performed.
- Ask how long the procedure will take.
- Ask how long the results are expected to last.

- Find about the extent of the recovery, overall healing, time out of work, etc.
- Ask to see pre and post-operative photographs of other patients he or she has worked on to get an idea of both his or her aesthetic skills and what results are reasonable for you to expect.
- Find out how many of the procedure(s) you are considering the doctor has done in the last month or the last year.

Choosing Where to Have Your Surgery

Cosmetic treatments and surgery can safely be performed in an accredited office-based surgical facility, a free-standing ambulatory surgicenter or in a hospital. For lesser procedures surgery can be arranged as an ambulatory or day case and you return home to complete your recovery. Outpatient surgical care has been proven to be safe, convenient and cost-effective, and can be performed in a variety of facilities. For major surgery that will be performed in a hospital, you may be admitted the evening before your operation, which is especially helpful if you live far from the hospital or clinic. In most cases you will be admitted on the day of surgery. For many cosmetic procedures performed in the U.S., it is common to go home the same day or within 24 hours. If your surgery will be performed outside of the hospital, check that your doctor has privileges to perform the same procedure in an accredited hospital. To research a hospital setting, contact the American Hospital Directory (www.ahd.com).

Accredited Facilities: To research a surgical center, find out who it is accredited by. Documentation of accreditation by one of the applicable governing bodies, the American Association for Accreditation of Ambulatory Surgery Facilities (AAAASF), the Accreditation Association for Ambulatory Health Care (AAAHC), or the Joint Commission on Accreditation of Healthcare Organizations (JCAHO), (appendix C) should be clearly visible in the location. Regulations for freestanding clinics and surgicenters fall under federal as well as state and local standards. More states will likely pass regulations covering office-based cosmetic surgery that will require doctors performing any cosmetic surgical procedure in an office-based facility to have privileges to perform the same procedure in an accredited hospital but this may not be the case in your particular state.

About Anesthesia

Modern anesthesia is safer than it has ever been due to safer drugs that affect body systems less and wear off more quickly after surgery as well as vastly improved monitoring equipment that allow a very careful watch on vital body functions. Methods of blocking pain sensation from specific areas of the face and body have improved so much in recent years that many minor cosmetic procedures can be done using some form of local anesthetic, with or without sedation. The anesthesiologist will ask if you want to be sleepy and relaxed before surgery. Some people prefer to be fully awake right up to induction of anesthesia. If you are particularly anxious the warm relaxing sensation of a sedative dose can relax you as the time for the operation draws nearer. It is also quite normal to be nervous as you try to fall asleep the night before your surgery. If you think you will need a sedative the night before surgery, your doctor may prescribe a single dose of medication to help you sleep.

Once you are wheeled into the operating room the anesthesiologist will begin by giving you a small injection that will make you feel drowsy. Within seconds you will be completely unconscious and that is usually the last thing you will remember of the actual procedure. If you will be under anesthesia for several hours, or are having extensive body surgery, you may have a rubber or plastic tube called a catheter inserted inside the urethra and into the bladder to keep your bladder empty during the surgery. The anesthetic will be supplied continuously to keep you comfortably asleep during the operation while a pulse oximeter, a device clipped onto your fingertip, will monitor your heart rate, EKG tracing, blood pressure, breathing rate, and the volume of gases you are breathing by the minute. The monitoring equipment used continuously checks your condition, especially the level of oxygen in your blood, and provides reliable surveillance so that the surgeon and anesthesiologist may be able to detect little problems at an early stage and make any necessary adjustments. If you are having only light sedation, it is possible that you will be able to mumble some words during surgery, but with general anesthesia you are in a very deep sleep. If you are moving about too much it will signal the anesthesiologist to give you more drugs to keep you comfortable and well sedated. You will have no recollection of being conscious or feeling any pain. The newest anesthetic agents work so quickly and efficiently that as soon as your IV goes in it will seem that you are waking up in the recovery room, astonished to find that the procedure is over.

Administering Anesthesia

You should inquire about the type of anesthesia you will be given, and, even more importantly, who will be administering it. The choice of the individual entrusted with providing your anesthesia is often not something you have control over, and it is sometimes not decided until the day before surgery. If you have particular concerns it is reasonable to ask to speak directly with the anesthesiologist in advance of surgery.

Anesthesiologist: Licensed physicians who complete a four-year college program, four years of graduate doctoral training and four years of anesthesiology residency. Anesthesiologists are the medical specialists who will immediately diagnose and treat any medical problems that might arise during your surgery or recovery period. If you are having general anesthesia, be sure your anesthesiologist is certified by the American Board of Anesthesiology - (919) 881-2570, www.abanes.org

PRE-ANESTHESIA QUESTIONS

- Is there is any chance you could be pregnant or are you nursing?
- What was the date of your last menstrual period?
- What medications are you currently taking?
- Have you or any family member had any problems with anesthesia?
- Do you have any allergies to medications?
- Are you a smoker?
- When was the last time you ate or drank?
- Do you bruise easily or have excessive bleeding from tooth extractions and menstrual cycles?

Certified Registered Nurse Anesthetist (CRNA): Licensed nursing professionals who have graduated from a nurse anesthesia educational program accredited by the Council on Accreditation of Nurse Anesthesia Educational Programs (COA). CRNAs may administer anesthesia for all types of surgical cases. American Association of Nurse Anesthetists - (847) 692-7050, www.aana.com. See Appendix C for more information.

Types of Anesthesia

Local: There is no loss of consciousness with local anesthesia, so patients are able to communicate with the physician and an anesthesiologist is usually not present. The local anesthetic agents temporarily prevent the nerves from carrying pain messages to the brain. The injection may be given directly into the area to be operated on or around the main trunks of the nerves that carry sensation. Another form of local anesthetic is a topical or surface form such as a spray, gel or cream applied to the area to be numbed. Some of these forms have to be left on the skin to penetrate for 30 minutes or longer before treatment.

Some of the procedures that local anesthesia is applicable for include botulinum toxin, dermal fillers, small liposuctions, non-ablative laser resur-

TYPE OF ANESTHESIA	TYPICAL APPLICATIONS
LOCAL	
	Botulinum toxin, dermal fillers, non-ablative laser resurfacing, small liposuctions, fat transfer, hair restoration, dental procedures
REGIONAL	
	Tummy tucks, calf implants, some lower body lifts and liposuction
TWILIGHT	
	Liposuction, eyelid surgery, ablative laser resurfacing, brow lifts, nasal surgery, breast lifts
GENERAL	
	Tummy tucks, body lifts, breast augmentation, breast reduction, bone grafts, nasal surgery, brow lifts

facing, fat transfer, hair restoration and dental procedures.

Regional: Regional anesthesia involves the injection of a local anesthetic to provide numbness, loss of pain or loss of sensation to a large region of the body. Regional anesthetic techniques include spinal blocks and epidural blocks that are usually supplemented with medications that will make you comfortable and drowsy.

Some of the procedures that regional anesthesia is applicable for include tummy tucks, calf implants, some lower body lifts and liposuction.

Twilight: (Monitored Anesthesia) Cosmetic procedures are often performed under local anesthesia with the addition of 'twilight' or a sedative given intravenously, such as Valium or Versed, so you can be thoroughly relaxed. These medications supplement local anesthetic injections, which are usually given by your cosmetic surgeon. You will be in a sleepy state, but may drift in and out of consciousness. This allows the direct area being operated on to be numbed, while you are relaxed, but not as heavily sedated as you would be with a general anesthesia.

Some of the procedures that twilight anesthesia is applicable for include liposuction, eyelid surgery, brow lifts, breast lifts, nasal surgery and ablative laser resurfacing.

General: A general anesthetic provides loss of consciousness and loss of sensation, and is commonly used in larger surgical procedures where the body may sustain a substantial amount of trauma, or if multiple procedures are being performed, or when it is necessary to turn the patient over. A general anesthetic is administered by injection, gas or a combination of both, and causes you to fall into a deep sleep. Other drugs are used to take away all sensations, to relax your muscles and to keep you from going into shock. The anesthesiologist puts you to sleep by giving you a small injection of rapidly acting and powerful drugs. Occasionally it is not possible to keep you comfortable with monitored or twilight anesthesia, so that general anesthesia may be needed.

Some of the procedures that general anesthesia is applicable to include tummy tuck, breast augmentation, breast reduction, body lifts, bone grafts, nasal surgery and brow lifts.

Anesthesia will affect your entire system so it is vital for your anesthesiologist to know as much about you as possible. If you do not meet your anesthesiologist during a preoperative interview, you will surely meet immediately before your surgery. The final clearance before surgery actually rests in the hands of the anesthesiologist who will review your medical chart to ensure that you are fit for surgery and that the anesthesia will be safe. If your blood pressure is elevated, or you have a chest infection or are running a slight fever or laboratory abnormalities, your surgery may be cancelled or postponed until you are well enough. Your anesthesiologist is responsible for managing medical problems that might arise related to surgery, as well as any chronic medical conditions you may have, such as asthma, diabetes, high blood pressure or heart problems.

"Aesthetic methodologies have increased dramatically; cosmetic surgery no longer offers just a few ways to get you there.

The Unofficial Guide™ *to Cosmetic Surgery (Macmillan, 1999)*
E. Bingo Wyer

WHAT HAPPENS BEFORE YOUR SURGERY

Before Surgery or Invasive Treatments

The fact that cosmetic treatments and surgery are generally performed on healthy people does not justify any lessening of customary standards of medical care; in fact, the standards should be even more stringent because it is elective. Before undergoing a surgical procedure you will be instructed to have a preoperative screening performed to pick up any potential contraindications to be dealt with before surgery such as anemia, clotting problems, positive Hepatitis B or C status, liver problems, diabetes, or hypertension. This process can be performed by your own primary care physician, at a lab, or at the hospital where your surgery will take place. The pre-surgical testing requirements for in-office surgery will be the same as if you were having surgery in a hospital setting. Generally, routine blood tests are required to be performed two weeks prior to surgery including CBC, SMA12, and PT/PTT. If you are age 40 and over, an EKG is usually required. For women of childbearing age, a BETA HCG or pregnancy test may also be requested. A chest x-ray may be ordered by the surgeon in individual cases as well, especially for smokers.

Additional testing may be ordered by the surgeon as needed for your specific case. For example, if you are having eyelid surgery, your surgeon may request that you undergo a Schirmer's Test to rule out a dry eye condition. If you are hav-

PRE-SURGICAL SCREENING
- General medical examination
- Height and weight
- Blood pressure measurement
- Urine analysis
- Blood analysis
- Chest x-ray
- Resting electrocardiogram (EKG)

ing difficulty breathing and planning to have nasal surgery, your surgeon may request that you have sinus x-rays. Before breast surgery a mammogram will often be requested or required. If you have a history of heavy menstrual periods, extreme bleeding, clotting disorders or excessive bruising, a Bleeding Time Test or evaluation by a hematologist may be ordered.

As a general rule, if you are under the care of a medical specialist for a particular condition and will be having anesthesia, it is a good idea to put your physician in touch with your specialist or request a letter of medical clearance for anesthesia and the proposed surgery.

Photography

Preoperative photographs usually will be required by the physician or dentist. Many doctors take their own photos using a digital camera in their offices. In some locations, like New York City, patients are referred to professional medical photographers for a special photo series prior to surgery. Typically, a series of six to ten shots will be taken so that the physician can view the area of the face or body from various angles. Preoperative photography is used as a road map or blueprint for the surgery: one doesn't look the same lying down as standing up. Even the trained eye of the cosmetic surgeon may often overlook imbalances and asymmetries. The photograph, however, is not subject to perceptual correction and shows everything, exactly as it is, to the doctor.

Preoperative photography is used as a road map or blueprint for the surgery: one doesn't look the same lying down as standing up.

Physicians generally prefer to use a solid background without harsh lighting and shadows. The standard photos needed are two lateral or side views, one from each side, two oblique or three-quarter views, one from each side, one frontal view and one view from the back. For rhinoplasty photos, a basal view showing the bottom of the nose is also necessary. Some doctors may also request photos with the patient smiling and at rest. These photographs will become part of your medical chart and they will be used to help plan your surgery. They also become a valuable tool for both you and your doctor to compare your final result. It is common to forget what your face, smile or body looked like before the surgery.

Having these photos or slides as documentation is a helpful reminder of the degree (or lack of) improvement you have achieved. Computer imaging is also frequently used by cosmetic doctors and dentists as a visual aid to show a prospective patient what may be achieved. New technologies such as 3-D computer imaging may also be used to help patients envision the results they may be able to expect. However, doctors cannot guarantee the computer-generated results you see on a screen. These should be used only as a guideline.

If you are contemplating a surgical procedure or treatment for the face, it is also helpful to the physician to bring in photographs of your face from approximately 10 years ago to see how you have changed. Facial rejuvenation techniques are often designed to bring the facial structures back to their former state.

chapter 9

"Beauty is the promise of happiness."

Henri B. Stendhal
1783-1842, French Writer

PREPARING FOR YOUR PROCEDURE

Having a pleasant cosmetic surgery experience is possible, but the key is in the planning. Scheduling a time when you can keep a low profile is often the most difficult part. Once you have determined when you will have your procedure, you will have a list of tasks to be completed.

Scheduling: There is no ideal season or time of year to undergo a cosmetic operation or treatment. This will vary depending on your lifestyle, work schedule, family commitments and personal preferences. For some people it is preferable to have procedures done in the colder months or wintertime. For others, their lives may slow down considerably during the summer, making that the only possible chance to recover in private. Holidays are always popular as well because it is easier to take time out of work. Because so many more people are considering cosmetic procedures, there is no longer a most popular time of year to have things done.

Smoking: Most surgeons will request, if not demand, that you stop smoking for two to three weeks prior to surgery. Nicotine constricts the blood vessels and can cause excessive bleeding and difficulty healing. "NO SMOKING" includes all forms of nicotine that infiltrate the bloodstream including patches, gum, tablets, chewing tobacco, cigars and pipes. If you cannot stop smoking altogether, limit yourself to as few cigarettes per day as possible. You will not be able to smoke the morning of surgery and for at least several days following surgery.

Medications: It is imperative that you tell your doctor about any and all medications you may be taking, by prescription and over the counter. You may be asked to give up alcohol, caffeine, aspirin and aspirin-containing drugs, hormone replacements or contraceptive pills and any other medications, including vitamins and supplements, that may cause blood clots and bruising. Do not take any medications that can thin your blood or disrupt the clotting process including Vitamin E, aspirin, ibuprofen, etc. Aspirin is a potent anticoagulant that can cause excessive bleeding. (See Appendix E for listing of medications.) You should not interrupt other medications you are taking unless your surgeon or anesthesiologist instructs you to; for example, for high blood pressure. If you are not sure what the active ingredients are in any supplements, vitamins, herbal teas and over-the-counter medications you are taking, bring them along in their original bottles for your anesthesiologist to evaluate. In some cases antibiotics will be prescribed to be taken prior to surgery; for example, for patients with a history of mitral valve prolapse, a heart murmur or previous hip or joint replacement.

> *Do not take any medications that can thin your blood or disrupt the clotting process including Vitamin E, aspirin, ibuprofen, etc.*

24 Hours Before Surgery: As a rule, you will be instructed not to eat or drink *anything* after midnight before your surgery, including water, coffee or tea. You will be instructed to brush your teeth the night before surgery or the morning of surgery without swallowing any water. If you wear dentures you should wear them to surgery. If you are having anesthesia (intravenous sedation or general), and you eat or drink within six to eight hours before, your procedure will be canceled or postponed. If you routinely take medications every morning and have been instructed to continue to do so, you will be told to take your pill(s) with a sip of water only.

What to Bring: On the morning of your procedure take a shower and DO NOT apply makeup, perfume, hair gels, moisturizers or any cosmetic to your face and/or body. Leave contact lenses home, but bring glasses if you have them. You should plan to wear only loose-fitting clothes that are easy to put on, button down the front, and will fit over bulky bandages or surgical dressings. Tight shoes, boots, and high heels are also not recommended, since your feet and ankles may swell after surgery and they will be hard to get on. Leave your valuables like jewelry and cash at home. If you are planning to spend the night in the hospital or surgicenter pack a small overnight bag with the bare essentials. An old nightgown or sweats, slippers or socks, a toothbrush and toothpaste and a change of clothes are all you really need. If you are having a facial procedure, sunglasses and a large scarf are helpful to cover up the next day. If your hair is very short you might want to let it grow out before surgery so that it is long enough to hide the scars around the ears and in the hairline while they heal. If your doctor has requested you to purchase a support bra or compression garment in advance, you may be asked to bring these with you. You do not need to bring along the prescriptions you have had filled prior to surgery, unless you will not be returning home after surgery.

"We can be beautiful at all ages. Feminine beauty comes in all shapes, sizes, colors, ways."

Lauren Hutton

THE RECOVERY PERIOD

After your surgery is completed you will be taken to the recovery room. For about the first 30 minutes you will be monitored by nursing staff. During this period you may be given extra oxygen and your breathing and heart functions will be observed closely. In some facilities you may then be moved to another area where you will continue to recover and family or friends may be allowed to be with you. You will be offered something to drink and you will be assisted in getting up. Nausea or vomiting may be related to anesthesia, the type of surgical procedure or postoperative pain medications. Medications to minimize postoperative pain, nausea and vomiting are usually given by your anesthesiologist during the surgical procedure and in recovery.

Depending on the policy of the hospital or surgicenter, and the type of surgery you had, most patients will be ready to go home between one to four hours after surgery. Occasionally it may be necessary to stay overnight or be transferred to a hospital if unanticipated side effects or complications occur. You must make arrangements for a responsible adult to take you home after your anesthetic or sedation. You will not be allowed to leave alone or drive yourself home. It is strongly suggested you have someone stay with you during the first 24 hours. If you have local anesthesia without sedation, it may be possible to go home without someone to accompany you.

For more extensive procedures, or if you live alone or prefer not to impose on family and friends, it may be suggested that you hire a private duty nurse to care for you for the first 24 - 48 hours. You will be able to walk slowly out of the hospital or clinic to a waiting car with some assistance. Once you are safely at home you should proceed directly to the room where you will be staying for most of the next 24 - 72 hours. It is best to rest in a room with a toilet and sink on the same floor to avoid having to walk up and down stairs. Change into a comfortable, loose-fitting nightgown, robe or sweats with necklines that do not pull over your head, and settle-in to rest. Wear skid-free socks or slippers if you have bare wood floors and stairs. Set up an extra few fluffy pillows in the bed for added comfort and, to avoid soiling, use waterproof pillow protectors. Rest inside, with moderate activity as tolerated for the first 48 hours, and avoid any strenuous physical exertion including driving, bending, carrying, lifting or exercise for a minimum of ten days. A stool softener may be recommended to avoid straining when going to the bathroom. Keep room temperature water at your bedside to swallow pills. You will be instructed on how to

POST-OP INSTRUCTIONS
24 Hours after surgery

- Do not drink any alcoholic beverages.
- Do not smoke or be in the presence of smokers.
- Avoid using the telephone, which can spread germs and cause infection.
- Do not take any medications, prescription or over the counter, unless instructed by your surgeon.
- Drink plenty of clear fluids; water, juice, broth.
- Eat a soft, bland diet as tolerated, working your way up to solid foods.
- Avoid salty, spicy, greasy foods, and preservatives.
- A bed tray can be helpful to serve meals.
- For facial surgery and some dental work, it may be easier to sip liquids through a straw.
- Never put ice packs directly on skin; wrap in soft washcloth or towel.
- Do not apply Vitamin E to your incision lines – it can cause allergic reactions.

keep your suture lines clean and dressings dry and intact, if you have any.

The amount of discomfort you experience will depend on many factors. You will be given pain medications by mouth or injection or by numbing the area around the incision. Your level of discomfort should be tolerable, but some amount of pain is to be expected. The more extensive the surgery, the greater amount of discomfort you will feel. For the first 24-48 hours after surgery you may need prescription pain medications. Most cosmetic surgeons will prescribe Tylenol with Codeine, Darvocet N100, or Vicodin ES. For more invasive surgery, such as abdominoplasty and breast reductions, something stronger may be given, like Percocet. After the first few days, most people switch to an over-the-counter pain medication or nothing at all.

You may experience drowsiness and minor after-effects following anesthesia, including muscle aches, a sore throat and occasional dizziness or headaches. Nausea may also occur, but vomiting is less common. These side effects usually decline rapidly in the hours following surgery, but it may take several days before they are gone completely. The majority of patients are not up to their usual routine for a few days until they feel back to normal. It is also normal to feel tired, anxious or depressed in the days or weeks following the operation. You will not look or feel like yourself immediately following surgery, but this is only a temporary condition. The period when you look your worst is typically at 72 hours or so. Your hormone levels change after surgery and you may start to feel sad or scared that you will never look like yourself again.

Keeping the head and torso elevated and applying cold compresses consistently will reduce swelling and relieve discomfort. Dressings should be kept dry and you will not be able to shower or bathe until your doctor allows it, which may be as early as one or two days. You may need some help with bathing and washing your hair. Avoid using water that is too hot or too cold; lukewarm or tepid water is best. Since you may be lightheaded for a few days after surgery, avoid getting up from a sitting position or out of bed too quickly. Keep one hand to steady yourself or ask for help if you feel dizzy. If you are having a face-lift, breast surgery or tummy tuck, drainage tubes may be required to prevent fluid collections. You will be instructed on how to empty your drains and record the amount of fluid so that your doctor can determine how long to keep them in place. Typically, drains are removed in a day or two, however in some cases up to a week may be necessary.

Generally, bruising resolves within the first three weeks following any cosmetic procedure. In some cases, there may be a slight discoloration or light bruising for longer if you have had excessive bleeding during surgery or post surgical complication that may delay

> **BASIC COSMETIC SURGERY RECOVERY TIMES–GENERAL GUIDELINES**
> - Back home: same day or next day
> - Shower: 1-2 days
> - Washing your hair: 1-2 days
> - Dressing removal: Next day
> - Suture removal: 3-7 days
> - Staple removal: 4-10 days
> - Surgical drain removal: 1-5 days
> - Aerobic exercise: 3-4 weeks
> - Bruising: up to 3 weeks
> - Makeup: 7-10 days

healing. The use of tissue glue or fibrin sealant intraoperatively may cut down on the amount of bruising and swelling that result. Camouflage makeup can usually be worn at about 10 days postoperatively to conceal discoloration, even around the eyelids. Exercise and sports can usually be resumed in three weeks. The initial swelling will resolve within the first few weeks, but may be present for several months or longer.

chapter 11

"There's a fine line between making a big improvement and having a fake, unnatural, and tight look. The bottom line is that if you decide to have any kind of plastic surgery, you cannot expect the end result to be perfect."

Beauty Evolution (Harper Collins, 2002)
by Bobbi Brown

CONSIDERING THE RISKS

It is a patient's right to be informed of the potential risks and complications of any medical procedure. Although your doctor or dentist will make every effort to minimize complications, it is not possible to eliminate the potential for all negative effects from occurring. With any medical or surgical procedure there is always a possibility of unexpected or unwanted events. No absolute guarantees as to the final result can ever be given by any physician. The ultimate decision to proceed rests with the patient, after the doctor has made a conscientious effort to explain every aspect of the procedure to the patient. Your doctor or dentist has a legal and ethical responsibility to explain these potential complications in detail so that you are well informed about what could go wrong and the attendant warning signs.

The risks of cosmetic surgery can be divided into two main groups: those that are common after all operations; and those that are unique to a specific technique or procedure. It is also important to factor in the variables of your individual health status, your age, skin quality, gender and your medical history. Clearly, a younger patient in prime health will have less risk than an older patient with a history of high blood pressure. Males are more prone to bleeding because they have a rich blood supply and thicker skin. Thin skinned patients may be more prone to bruising. The most common risks of cosmetic procedures include swelling, bruising, bleeding, infection, prolonged numbness and a reaction to anesthesia. General surgical complications may include hematoma, which is a blood clot; seroma, which is a collection of clear fluid; nerve damage, scar tissue formation, asymmetries and irregularities. Infections are rare and are typically treated with a course of antibiotics. It is common to be prescribed an antibiotic before and/or after surgery to guard against infection. If you are having a surgery that involves placing an implant or graft, there is always the possibility of extrusion, whereby the implant works its way up to the surface of the skin, and capsular contracture, which is an excess tightening of scar tissue that forms around the implant.

Most Common Risks & Complications of Cosmetic Procedures

General Risks

- Hematoma
- Seroma
- Skin sloughing (skin loss)
- Nerve damage (temporary injury to a nerve)
- Infection
- Bleeding
- Delayed healing
- Poor scarring or keloids (raised or hypertrophic scars)
- Prolonged numbness
- Reaction to anesthesia or medications (allergic reaction, nausea, vomiting)

Serious Complications

- Pulmonary embolus (a blood clot)
- Fat embolus
- Permanent nerve damage
- Malignant hyperthermia
- Arrhythmia
- Sepsis
- Death

If you have a history of bad scarring or thickened scars, such as keloids, or delayed healing from past surgical procedures, you should inform your physician ahead of time. In general, the immediate scars will remain somewhat thickened and red for weeks and often months, then gradually become less obvious, ideally eventually fading to thin white lines. Smoking can increase the risks of this procedure because nicotine constricts the blood vessels, decreases blood flow to tissues and greatly increases the chance of scarring. In some cases, smokers can actually lose a portion of skin due to decreased oxygen flow into the skin caused by carbon monoxide. Nicotine substitutes and smoker's aids, can also increase the risk of poor healing, skin sloughing, scabbing and crusting. These risks are significantly reduced if you stop smoking at least two weeks before surgery and wait until you are completely healed before starting again, or preferably quit smoking entirely. However, even if you exercise these precautions there is no guarantee.

In some cases, smokers can actually lose a portion of skin due to decreased oxygen flow into the skin caused by carbon monoxide.

After the procedure you will be instructed to be on the lookout for the signs of infection near the incisions: increased swelling, redness, high fever, warmth, bleeding, or other discharge. You'll be asked to check that your bowels are functioning normally since constipation is common. If you experience any unusual symptoms, such as heavy bleeding, throbbing, or sudden pain followed by significant swelling, report them to your doctor or dentist right away.

In the following chapters you will find a detailed description of many of the most common potential complications specific to each treatment covered in this guide.

chapter 12

"If you consult a surgeon who agrees with everything you want, one who will nip, and tuck and pull anything, without hesitation or concern, run for your life."

Making Faces (Little, Brown and Company, 1997)
by Kevin Aucoin.

COSTS

Fees for cosmetic surgery vary widely depending on the extent of the procedure, the number of procedures being done in one stage, the amount of time it will take to perform, the geographic region you are having it performed in and, of course, the surgeon you select. For example, fees are higher in major metropolitan areas like New York City and Los Angeles than in a small suburban town. It is never wise to choose a doctor for a cosmetic procedure solely on the basis of cost. When calculating the total costs, there are several separate charges to consider. First, there is the doctor's fee. There may be the additional cost of an operating room and for the anesthesiologist if one is required. The operating facility also may bill for laboratory and for supplies separately. Fees quoted should be all inclusive. Ask for a breakdown so you understand all of the costs involved. Some doctors will apply the consultation fee you have paid towards the cost of your procedure. The anesthesiologist's fee may be set at a fixed amount or a percentage of the surgical fee, or it may be charged based on the number of hours the surgery takes.

ITEMIZED COSTS

- Consultation fee
- Surgical fee
- Deposit
- Anesthesia fee
- Hospital or Operating Room charges
- Photography
- Medications
- Laboratory fees
- Implants
- Supplies and dressings
- Surgical garments
- Nursing Care

Consultation

Most doctors will charge a consultation fee that is paid on the day of your initial visit. In some cases, this fee may be applied to the cost of the procedure you are having. Consultations may range from $75 to $350 in special cases. Many doctors today also offer consultations via their website, which is especially helpful for out of town patients.

Deposits

It is common in cosmetic procedures for fees to be paid in advance. Many doctors will require a non-refundable deposit to hold a surgical date, which can vary from a nominal amount like $500.00 to ten or twenty-five percent or more of the total fee. If you cancel surgery without adequate notice, many doctors will charge a cancellation fee or retain a percentage of your deposit. The balance of the fee is often due two to four weeks prior to the date of your procedure. Most doctors' offices accept several methods of payment, including personal checks, cash and major credit cards. Some also participate in financing programs to help you finance the cost of surgery over time.

Surgical Revisions

You should also inquire about the doctor or dentist's policy on additional surgery or revisions. If you are not entirely satisfied with your result, find out what options you may have and what can be done. If your doctor stands behind his or her work, he may be willing to do a revision at no additional charge, or a small charge, within a certain amount of time, such as six months to one year. You will most likely be required to pay for the cost of the facility and anesthesia. Fortunately, most poor surgical outcomes can be improved, at least to some degree. Know in advance what kind of recourse you might have.

Insurance

Cosmetic surgery is considered elective and is, therefore, usually not covered by health insurance plans. Some operations, such as breast reduction or rhinoplasty, may have a functional component that may fall under the domain of reconstructive surgery. In these cases, your insurance company may cover part or all of the surgery fee, the anesthesia fee and the hospital expenses. In order to qualify for insurance coverage it is recommended that you contact your plan in advance to determine the specific criteria.

Cost table

The following table is from The American Society
for Aesthetic Plastic Surgery (ASAPS)

Procedure	Physician/Surgeon Fees*
Abdominoplasty (tummy tuck)	$4,477
Botulinum Toxin Injections (Botox®,Myobloc®)	$413
Breast Augmentation	$3,257
Breast Lift	$4,616
Breast Reduction	$5,183
Buttock Lift	$4,616
Cellulite Treatment (mechanical roller massage therapy)	$503
Cheek Implants	$2,376
Chemical Peel (ranges from light to deep)	$831
Chin Augmentation	$1,735
Collagen Injection	$350
Dermabrasion	$1,367
Ear Surgery	$2,589
Eyelid Surgery	$2,510
Face-Lift	$5,622
Fat Injection	$1,065
Forehead Lift	$2,779
Gynecomastia Treatment of	$2,894
Hair Transplantation	$3,580
Laser Hair Removal	$423
Laser Skin Resurfacing	$2,250
Laser Treatment of Leg Veins	$427
Lip Augmentation (surgical)	$1,487
Lipoplasty (liposuction)	$2,425
Lower Body Lift	$5,833
Microdermabrasion	$201
Rhinoplasty	$3,745
Sclerotherapy	$273
Thigh Lift	$4,078
Upper Arm Lift	$3,056

* National average; surgeon fees vary considerably by geographic region. Facility fees, anesthesia and other surgical costs not included.

Financing Cosmetic Surgery and Treatment

Cosmetic surgery and cosmetic dentistry can be expensive. As the chart on the facing page demonstrates, if multiple procedures are preformed total costs can range from a few thousand dollars to tens of thousands, especially when costs for anesthesia, facility fees and others are included.

Since very little of cosmetic care is covered by insurance, most people pay "out of pocket". However, that doesn't mean that someone should not pursue reimbursement from their health plan for cosmetic care. Some procedures may be covered. A rhinoplasty, for example, may correct a breathing problem as well as improve ones appearance. A blepharoplasty may remove bags that are impairing one's vision and, thus, may be eligible for coverage. Despite these examples and others, the reality is that most people will have to pay for cosmetic care themselves. As a result, there are a number of companies that have been created to help consumers finance these costs.

Just hearing about a low interest rate is not enough to assess the costs of the loan. You must calculate the total payments, month by month, to understand what the loan and the procedure will really cost. Like any loan, the borrower has to look carefully at the fine print. The contract must be examined for extra payments, late fees, pre-payments, pre-payment penalties and all the other elements of any loan agreement. If you do not have experience in taking out a loan ask a lawyer, accountant, or even an experienced relative or friend to review the loan agreement for you.

Some financing companies pre-qualify you for a loan and then send you a list of "approved" doctors who participate in their program. These doctors typically pay a fee to be part of these networks and there is no screening of the doctors involved. The doctors and dentists who agree to participate are "approved"; but only by the loan company. That doesn't mean they are not qualified, only that you need to screen them as you would any other physician or dentist. It is very important to choose a competent well-trained physician or dentist for cosmetic care. That is the most important decision. The method of financing your care should be secondary to that.

chapter 13

*"The question is: how do you know that you're in the right hands?
Ultimately, it's your decision, and for that, you have to do research.
This is one instance when listening to your best friend is not enough."*

How To Be Beautiful: The Thinking Woman's Guide (Random House, 2002)
by Kathleen Baird-Murray.

SECOND OPINIONS

There is no precise formula for choosing the right physician or dentist for
cosmetic procedures. Ultimately, you have to use your own judgment
and instincts. Never go with the first or only doctor you see; always get
at least a second opinion and preferably three or more before you
choose. Even if you may love the first doctor you see and feel very comfortable with him, see at least one or two others for confirmation and
comparison. After the third, you may still find you want to go with the
first one you visited, but only after you see others are you really qualified to choose wisely. Unless you feel comfortable with the doctor and
what he or she is recommending for you, wait and re-think it, or see
another doctor until it feels like a good fit. If it doesn't feel right, you
should always continue with the interview process. You need not feel
that you have made a commitment to a doctor or dentist after having had
a single consultation. Once you have narrowed down your list to two or
three names, go back and see the front-runner again. You should always
see the doctor or dentist who will be doing your actual procedure at least
twice before the operation. The initial consultation may be with a nurse,
receptionist or office manager; however, the evaluation should be with
the doctor or dentist to be performing the procedure. The next visit is
normally scheduled closer to the date of your treatment so you will have
an opportunity to ask any questions you may have forgotten to ask the
first time. This second meeting should leave you feeling confident that
you have made a wise choice. You may still have some sleepless nights
and pre-surgery jitters but, by this time, you should have confidence in
the doctor you have chosen.

Finding the right cosmetic doctor or dentist is a very personal journey. What appeals to one person may be totally inappropriate or offensive to another. You owe it to yourself to approach any cosmetic procedure as an empowered and educated consumer.

section

II

SURGERY OF THE FACE

Whether you accept it or not, we live in a society where looks count. How you feel about the way you look sends off a signal to the world that you are confident, successful and content. All of us have one or several flaws that we would love to improve. It may be the bump on your nose, the fatty bags beneath your eyes, ears that stick out, or a weak chin. Fortunately, modern advances in cosmetic surgery and dentistry have made it possible to enhance your appearance safely, effectively and with less pain, bruising and recovery time than a decade ago. A common misconception of cosmetic surgery is that once you have a face-lift, you'll have to keep having them. In fact, the opposite is true. If you ask how long a face-lift will last, the answer is forever. You will always look better for having had a lift at whatever stage you do it. As the face continually changes with age, the benefits of having undergone surgery will ensure that you will look younger than your chronological age. Cosmetic surgery of the face involves far more than just the basic face-lift. In the following section you will find comprehensive descriptions and pertinent details about all of the most popular techniques for the face, eyes, brow, nose and ears. Many of these procedures may be combined in one stage or performed in several stages. It is tempting to do a few procedures at once or close together, but it is not always practical. Once you've healed, you might not be willing to undertake another procedure within a few months or even years. Cosmetic enhancements can be very seductive, but surgery should never be looked on as a fashion statement, fad or craze. Each procedure should be given careful consideration, especially if it is being undertaken to change a facial feature or make you look different.

Eyelid surgeries jumped 91 percent between 1992 and 2002, and the procedure ranked sixth overall for people having cosmetic surgery.

American Society of Plastic Surgeons

THE EYES

Blepharoplasty (Eyelid Surgery)

Eyelid skin lacks the requisite tone-retaining muscles and oil content, which leaves it more prone to wrinkling. The eyelids age in a couple of ways. Sun exposure without the protection of sunglasses will have a direct effect on the weakening of your elastic fibers that keep eyelid skin taut. Droopy eyelids, or puffy lower eyelids, often run in families and are as common in men as in women. Protruding fatty tissue from your eye sockets that causes bags can be an inherited trait that shows up early in life, as well as the result of aging. At first bags, or sagging, may be most noticeable when you are particularly tired; then the signs become visible all of the time. Eyelid skin thins and stretches as it ages, becomes loose and, with time, muscles weaken and fat that cushions the eyeball moves forward around the eyes. Puffiness results when a fat pad that cushions the eye begins to pull away from the bone of the lower eye and sags. Gravity has its effects on the eyes as well. Sagging upper eyelids may result in hooding over the eyes where upper lids become heavier and fuller. Eyelid surgery should never compromise the functional elements of the eyelids for the sake of aesthetics. Blepharoplasty can reduce droopy or hooded eyelids, restore the contour to the lids and eliminate the protruding fat bags under the eyes. In some cases eyelid surgery may also correct severe hooding of the upper eyelids called 'ptosis', which can obstruct peripheral vision and reduce the range of upward vision.

Surgical Methods

In blepharoplasty, excess fat, skin and, if needed, muscle are removed from the upper and/or lower eyelids. The procedure is usually performed on an outpatient basis under local anesthesia with intravenous sedation. First, eye drops may be used to anesthetize the eyes and then protective contact lenses may be placed over the eyes during the surgery. Sometimes a laser may also be used as a cutting tool to make the incision and to remove excess fat. Very fine electrocautery is used throughout eyelid surgery to minimize bleeding.

Lower Eyelids: The incision typically extends into the crow's feet where lines already exist so that the scar will be less noticeable. The most common methods of performing lower blepharoplasty are the traditional approach, sometimes called a skin-muscle flap, and the transconjunctival approach. For the traditional approach, an incision is made adjacent to the lower lashes to be as inconspicuous as possible. The surgeon lifts the skin and muscle to remove a small amount of fat. Excess skin and muscle are then trimmed from the lower lid. If you have a pocket of fat beneath your lower eyelids, but do not have any loose skin, your surgeon may recommend a transconjunctival blepharoplasty. It is usually performed on younger patients with fatty lower eyelids and elastic skin. The transconjunctival method utilizes an incision hidden inside the lower eyelid that leaves no visible external scars. Through this incision the surgeon exposes and trims the excess fat. The incision is closed with self-dissolving sutures or, more commonly, it is left to heal on its own. A lid tightening procedure may also be performed at the same time if there is muscle laxity, or may be reserved for a later stage. Transconjunctival techniques are particularly advantageous for men because there is no visible scar. The transconjunctival is the less invasive and a traditional skin-muscle flap can always be done at a future date when it becomes necessary. It is quite common to combine resurfacing with Carbon Dioxide or Erbium:YAG lasers or a trichloracetic acid peel (TCA) at the same time as a transconjunctival blepharoplasty. The laser or peel has the effect of a slight tightening and smoothing of any loose skin that may remain after the fat bags are removed. Another aspect of lower eyelid surgery is the formation of "tear troughs", deep grooves that can result when there is an obvious demarcation between where the lower eyelid area ends and the cheek begins. The main methods used to address this are fat transposition, where

> *The transconjunctival method utilizes an incision hidden inside the lower eyelid that leaves no visible external scars.*

the fatty deposits are moved around to create a smoother look, fat removal or fat replacement.

Upper Eyelids: Upper eyelid blepharoplasty involves making an elliptical incision across the eyelid crease in the natural skin fold. This is done by finding the edge of the tarsal plate, the supporting cartilage of the upper eyelid. The surgeon draws a line to identify the lower edge of the skin that will be excised, which will eventually become the scar that remains. The excess skin of the upper eyelid is then marked out. Excess skin and fatty tissue are removed along with a thin strip of muscle to give the eyelid crease more definition. The incision is then closed with a single layer of sutures, usually hiding the scar within the natural fold of the upper eyelids. It is common to use a single long stitch, called a running stitch, on the upper eyelid. In some cases a transconjunctival approach may be used for the upper eyelids as well. This procedure leaves no visible scar and a small amount of fat may be removed from the inside of the upper eyelid. Fatty deposits will tend to recur over time. After traditional upper eyelid surgery residual fat in the inner corners of the eyelids may be removed at a future date if needed via a transconjunctival approach.

Operating Time: 1-3 hours

The Recovery Period

Thin sterile bandages will be applied to the incisions after the surgery. An ointment to prevent dryness may be applied, but it is not necessary for the eyes to be covered. Depending on the extent of your procedure some swelling and bruising is to be expected for several weeks. Keeping your head elevated with extra pillows above the level of your heart when lying down can help speed up healing. Applying cold compresses or ice packs for the first 48 hours will reduce swelling. Your eyelids will feel tight and sore as the anesthesia wears off. You can also expect to feel a slight burning sensation. Fine sutures used to close the incision are removed three to five days after the procedure. Although you will be able to read, use a computer and watch television after a few days, these activities should be limited because your eyes will feel easily tired and these activities tend to dry the eyes. For seven to ten days the eye area will need to be cleaned and the eyes may feel sticky and itchy. In some cases your surgeon will recommend using eye drops. Contact lenses should not be worn for one to two weeks and may feel uncomfortable for a while when you resume wearing them. Excessive blinking, which leads to increased swelling, also should be avoided if possible. Avoid drinking alcohol, which dries out the eyes, causes fluid retention and can prolong recovery. Sunglasses should be worn because the eye area will be sensitive to sun, wind, and other irritants for several weeks. For the first two weeks avoid any activity that increases blood flow to the eyes, including bending, lifting, crying and exercise or sports. Although your scars can remain slightly pink for six months after surgery, they should eventually fade to a thin, barely visible white line. Eyelid scars heal well because of the thinness of the skin and rarely form keloids.

Back to Work: 7-10 days

Potential Risks or Side Effects

Certain medical conditions, including dry eyes or lack of sufficient tears, thyroid problems like hypothyroidism and Graves' disease, hypertension, cardiovascular disease, and diabetes may increase the risks associated with eyelid surgery. Before surgery your surgeon may require an examination by an ophthalmologist to perform glaucoma testing and measure tear production. A dry eye condition, or blepharitis, can inhibit healing and possibly result in injury or infection of the cornea. Your ophthalmologist may recommend against surgery if your dry eye condition is very severe, or choose a more conservative surgical approach. In some cases, an additional procedure to tighten the lower eyelid horizontally may be required. Minor complications may include temporary double or blurred vision for a few days, burning, stinging, gritty sensation in the eye, excessive tearing, and a slight asymmetry. Tiny whiteheads or milia may appear after the sutures are removed. They can be easily removed by your surgeon. Severe complications may include decreased sensation in the eyelid, dry eyes, difficulty closing eyes completely, prominent or hardened scars, or an ectropion, where the lower lid is pulled down. A more serious, but rare, complication is bleeding behind the eye, called a retrobulbar hematoma.

Alternative Treatment Options

The goals of eyelid rejuvenation techniques are to remove excess skin and fat, to re-establish the crease in the upper lids, and to correct slack muscles that pull the lower lid down. Eyelid surgery does not correct dark circles under the eyes or fine lines and wrinkles. Dark circles are often a vascular problem caused by dilated blood vessels under the eyes, or by dark pigmentation or very thin skin. Surgery of the eyelids will also not lift sagging eyebrows, which requires a brow or forehead lift that can be performed in tandem with eyelid surgery. Laser resurfacing, chemical peels or botulinum toxin injections can reduce fine lines and wrinkles near the eye. Eyelid surgery may be repeated as needed, but tends to last many years, from five to ten or more.

Surgical Fee: $2,000 - $5,000; there may be additional fees for the hospital, surgicenter, and anesthesia. Some eyelid surgery may fall within the realm of medical necessity, especially when excess skin overhangs part of the eye and interferes with your field of vision. This is more common on older people over age 65.

The Brow

As the skin ages, it begins to lose its elasticity resulting in frown lines, wrinkling across the forehead and an increasing heaviness that pulls the eyebrows down. Forehead lifts are an option if you have a sagging brow or deep furrows between the eyes. A forehead or brow lift tightens loose skin and in, some cases, removes the excess skin, and forehead wrinkling and drooping brows can be modified. When necessary, part of the muscle that causes vertical frown lines between the brows is also removed. Although the skin may be tightened, scars, age spots, fine lines and creases will soon return to their original texture. Skin treatments like laser skin resurfacing and chemical peels can improve the texture of the skin and are frequently used in combination with a forehead lift. Finally botulinum toxin injections can retard the formation of wrinkles. Dermal fillers are sometimes used with botulinum toxin to plump out the glabellar creases that forms between the eyebrows.

Surgical Methods

There are two basic techniques used; the more traditional coronal brow lift and variations of an endoscopic forehead lift. For a coronal brow lift the incision is made slightly behind the natural hairline, running from ear to ear across the top of the head, in the same place that a hair band, or headset, would sit. The incision is usually made well behind the hairline so that the scar is not visible. If your hairline is high or receding, the incision may be placed just at the hairline, so as not to move the forehead back. In patients who are losing hair a mid-scalp incision that follows the natural pattern of the skull bones may be preferred. Wearing bangs over your forehead will usually conceal the scars sufficiently. The endoscopic forehead lift typically requires the same preparation as the coronal browlift procedure, but offers the advantages of minimal incisions within the scalp and a potentially shorter recovery period.

An endoscope, a small wand with a camera on the end connected to a monitor, is inserted to allow the surgeon to have a clear view of the muscles and tissues beneath the skin.

Coronal Lift: Most forehead lifts are performed under local anesthesia combined with a sedative to make you drowsy. This keeps you in a twilight state and you'll be relaxed, and unable to feel pain. Some surgeons prefer to use general anesthesia. To begin, your hair is tied back with rubber bands on either side of your head where the incision will be made. The head does not need to be shaved. After the incision is made the skin of the forehead is lifted away from the underlying tissue so that it can be removed and the muscles of the forehead can be released. The eyebrows may also be elevated and excess skin is trimmed away. The incision is then closed with stitches or staples. Most surgeons do not use any dressings, but some may cover the incision with gauze padding and wrap the head in an elastic bandage.

Endoscopic Brow lift: Rather than making one long incision, the surgeon makes between three to five scalp incisions of approximately one inch in length. An endoscope, a small wand with a camera on the end connected to a monitor, is inserted to allow the surgeon to have a clear view of the muscles and tissues beneath the skin. Another instrument is then inserted through a different incision, the forehead skin is lifted and the muscles and underlying tissues are removed or released. The eyebrows may also be lifted and secured into their higher position by sutures beneath the surface of the skin or by temporary fixation screws and other methods placed behind the hairline. Finally, the incisions are closed with stitches or staples. Gauze and an elastic bandage may also be used, but is not always necessary.

The Recovery Period

You will be instructed to keep your head elevated and apply cold compresses to reduce swelling. Any bandages are removed within a few days after surgery. Stitches or staples are removed within a week and the temporary fixation screws or other materials within two weeks. You will be able to shower and shampoo your hair within a couple of days or when the bandage is removed. There may be numbness and temporary pulling around the incision. If you are prone to headaches you may be treated with an additional longer-acting local anesthesia during surgery as a preventive measure. Swelling and bruising may also affect the cheeks and eyes but should begin to disappear in a week or so. As the nerves heal, the scalp may begin to itch, which may continue for up to six months. Some of the hair around the incision may thin out, but normal growth usually resumes within a few weeks to several months. Although you should be up and about in a few days, plan on resting for at least the first week after surgery. Rigorous physical activity including jogging, bending, heavy lifting, and sex, should be limited for several weeks. Most of the visible signs of surgery should fade within the first three weeks.

Back to Work: 7-10 days

Potential Risks or Side Effects

If a complication arises during an endoscopic forehead lift the surgeon may abandon this technique and switch to the coronal procedure, which will result in a more extensive scar. There is a possibility that the nerves that control brow movement may be injured on one or both sides, which may result in an inability to raise the eyebrows or wrinkle the forehead. This is usually a temporary condition, but may be long term or permanent in rare cases. Another potential complication is the formation of a widened scar, which may require another surgical procedure to create a new, thinner scar. The loss of sensation along or just beyond the incision line is common, especially with the coronal brow lift. Numbness is usually temporary and will resolve in three to four months.

Alternative Treatment Options

Skin type, ethnic background, degree of skin elasticity, individual healing, basic bone structure, all should be discussed prior to surgery. Less invasive procedures may be alternatives, but they cannot always produce the same results.

Surgical Fee: $2,500-$5,000, there may be additional fees for the hospital, surgicenter and anesthesia

"In some of the wealthiest circles, there is the dress by the couturier, and the face by the elite and well-known surgeon, and the body by the high-ticket personal trainer."

Survival of the Prettiest (Abacus, 1999)
by Nancy Etcoff

The Face

The face-lift, as well as the facial rejuvenation procedures that are commonly performed with it (eyelid surgery and brow lifts), remain the only viable option to restore a youthful appearance when the lower face and neck have begun their inevitable descent. There is no such thing as a perfect or ideal face-lift. Skin type, ethnic background, degree of skin elasticity, individual healing and basic bone structure all factor into your options. A face-lift can tighten loose skin and muscle and remove or reposition excess fat to eliminate sagging. The most significant degree of improvement is usually seen in the jowls, lower face and neck. No two faces age alike and all the anatomical components of facial aging do not change at exactly the same pace. Reversal of facial aging is not achieved through surgical rearrangement of the deep tissues and skin excision alone. Face-lift procedures are constantly changing and the actual concept of facial rejuvenation has evolved to encompass more of a remodeling, not just pulling skin more taut. Facial shaping by removing, repositioning or adding soft tissue, rather than by tightening the skin and muscles alone, is considered the key to achieving optimal results in facial rejuvenation. Some people will only have one face-lift in their lifetime. Others may have a second surgery five to ten years later when the tissues have relaxed again. There is no specific limit of how many facelifts any one person may have, and it is not uncommon to have more than one in a lifetime.

Surgical Methods

Face-lift surgery can be performed under local anesthesia with sedation or general anesthesia. Your hair will be held back with rubber bands during surgery, but the hair does not need to be shaved. Traditional face-lift incisions generally start above the hairline at the temples and continue along a line in front of the ear or just inside the cartilage at the front of the ear, behind the earlobe and back into the scalp. Another small incision is often made under the chin to address the neck. The surgeon separates the skin from the underlying fat and muscle. The underlying muscle fascia is tightened along with the platysma muscle in the neck and excess fat is removed. After the deep tissues are tightened, the excess skin is pulled up

MOST COMMON FACE-LIFT TECHNIQUES

SMAS LIFT. Excess skin is removed and redraped, the skin and the SMAS, or underlying muscle layer, are elevated and tightened, fatty tissue under the neck is suctioned.

EXTENDED SMAS LIFT. Excess skin is removed and redraped, underlying muscle layer is freed from the cheek ligaments, and more tension is placed on the muscle layer instead of skin flap.

SUBPERIOSTEAL LIFT. This lift can be done with the aid of an endoscope and/or via an incision running horizontally across the scalp with or without incisions placed inside the mouth used to free the fat, muscle and skin layers off the bone so they can be pulled up and tightened.

COMPOSITE LIFT. This lift is also referred to as a "Deep Plane Face-lift", a total facial rejuvenation including the upper and lower eyelids, usually an open brow lift, face and neck; the facial tissues, fat, muscles and skin are lifted in one continuous section. Deeper face-lifts tend to be more invasive than conventional methods and may produce more prolonged swelling.

MID FACE-LIFT. This lift is also referred to as a "Cheek Lift" that addresses the triangular shaped section of the middle of the face. This technique does not usually improve the neck or lower face and may be combined with a neck lift procedure.

and back and then trimmed. The incisions are closed with stitches and/or staples on the scalp. A dressing is applied to protect the entire area. Most people can return home after the surgery or stay in a nearby hotel for the first night. Some choose to remain in the hospital or in a recovery facility for a day or more.

The SMAS-lift is still considered the most commonly performed face-lift technique today. In addition to the skin flap face-lift and SMAS technique, there has been a proliferation of new techniques and variations on older methods. Each of these methods has its proponents, but it has yet to be conclusively demonstrated that any one technique is greatly superior for every patient. No single formula is right for everyone; the surgical plan must be customized for each individual patient. Sometimes the glands in the neck underneath the chin may be very prominent and need to be removed or repositioned during a face-lift. The traditional face-lift operation requires a continual incision that starts two to three inches above the ear in the temple, then down in front of the ear for two to three inches around and into the crease behind the ear with an extension into the hair behind the ear, which adds up to about eight inches in most people. The modified techniques may cut the scar down to three or four inches in total, usually reducing the scar that extends behind the ear. A modified face-lift, also referred to as a "minimal" or "mini"-face-lift, or in some circles an 'S-Lift", is a good option for younger patients who do not require as much correction. It is less invasive which translates to reduced swelling, scarring, bruising and risk. The ideal patient for an extended mini-face-lift is someone who has looked good up until recently and is now beginning to get comments like, "You're looking tired." The end result replaces anatomic structures where they once resided without changing the patient's look significantly.

Some of the newest methods are innovative in the length and positioning of the scars. Instead of making an incision into the hairline in two places, the newer methods stop before the incision gets into the hairline. The incisions that tend to cause the most problems lie in the crease behind the ear and in the hair, and this procedure eliminates most of those. Even a few days less healing time can make a difference between being able to have a face-lift in the narrow window of time you can set aside and having to put it off for a year or two. Modified or limited incision lifts have the advantage of a shorter recovery and can be applied to different scenarios including men. In general, you will have a better and more natural result at a younger age when the signs of aging are just beginning to appear but are not full blown. The end result is a refreshed appearance rather than waiting till they start looking old and need surgery to make them look younger again.

Operating Time: 2-6 hours depending on the technique used and the extent of the procedure

The Recovery Period

Your entire face and neck may be bandaged to minimize bruising and swelling. To drain any blood that might collect a small tube may be inserted under the skin behind your ear for a day or two. Keep your head elevated, above heart level when lying down. Your surgeon will advise that you rest for 72 hours and to avoid placing added tension on the scars. There is some discomfort for several days after surgery and you will be given a prescription for medication to alleviate it. Severe

> *Some tightness and numbness of the skin can be expected that will resolve in a few weeks to months.*

pain is unusual and should be a warning sign to alert your doctor. Cold compresses will help reduce swelling and soothe pain. Dressings are usually removed within one to five days and most stitches can be removed after five to ten days. Once the bandages are removed you can shower and gently shampoo your hair. The hair around your temples may be thin at first, but normally grows back in four months. It is important to stay away from alcohol, steam baths and saunas for several weeks. Your scalp may take longer to heal and scars will be red at first, fading to pink and may take up to a year to fade to white lines. Some tightness and numbness of the skin can be expected that will resolve in a few weeks to months. You may look pale, bruised and quite swollen at first, but in a few weeks the effects become more visible. It is common to have areas of hardness, especially around the chin and neck, from swelling and lumps and bumps may form in the cheeks during the healing process. Strenuous activities like heavy lifting and rigorous exercise should be avoided for at least two weeks. It is not uncommon to feel a bit depressed because facial features may be distorted from the swelling, facial movements may be slightly stiff and the bruising and scarring can make you self-conscious. Major social engagements should be postponed for four to six weeks until you feel comfortable with your new look.

Back to Work: 10-14 days

Potential Risks or Side Effects

Drainage may be required for prevent hematomas. If that occurs, the patient must return to the doctor's office or operating room where the surgeon will open the incision line and remove the excess fluid collected. Injury to the nerves that control facial muscles is a potential serious complication. Most postoperative numbness is only temporary. Skin sloughing around the incisions is another complication that may occur, especially in smokers. Poor or delayed healing of the skin may also occur in people who have very thin skin, most likely in the neck behind the ear where the most tension is placed during closure. Thickened or raised scars are a possible consequence of face-lift surgery, but can be treated by surgical revision, laser therapy and steroid injections if necessary. A small shift in the position of the hairline is common, but if you started out with an elevated hairline this can be an unwanted side effect. Informing your surgeon about how you wear your hair is a good idea so that he or she can plan his incisions accordingly to avoid any potential scarring that may be a problem if you plan to resume wearing your hair short or off your neck.

Alternative Treatment Options

Cosmetic surgeons can approach the neck in several ways, but if jowls and loose skin are the chief concern a surgical procedure will be recommended. The most important factor is whether your aging neck is related to the skin and/or musculature. On a younger neck with good skin quality unwanted fat in the neck and jowl areas can be suctioned. This procedure can give the neck a sharper line and better contour. Liposuction alone works best on young, toned skin that is elastic and will shrink back after the fatty deposits are removed. When just the fat is removed, muscle bands may appear more prominent after the cushiony fatty tissue that was camouflaging these structures is removed. Similarly, neck flaws are easier to spot in a thin neck. The key is in the quality and quantity of the skin. If you have loose skin, or a "turkey gobbler" neck to start with, a more extensive procedure is probably indicated. If you don't want a complete face-lift, and you have minimal loose skin and platysma bands, a platysmaplasty may be performed by sewing the muscle bands together through an incision under the neck with a suture suspension technique. A neck lift can also be done endoscopically alone, or in addition to other work on the upper face. This method allows for excess fat to be removed that rests above and/or below the muscle in the neck, and/or tightening of the neck muscles, usually without skin removal. If the skin is very slack, a lower face-lift will give better control in most patients. Botulinum toxin is frequently used in the neck to soften the muscle bands, but will not significantly improve jowls or tighten loose skin. A face-lift can soften, but not totally eliminate the creases between your nose and the corners of your mouth. Face-lifts mainly address the lower two thirds of the face and the neck, but do little to improve the eye and brow area unless the operation is specifically designed to address aging of the upper face. Consequently, face-lifts are often done in conjunction with other procedures including laser resurfacing, eyelid surgery, brow lifts, botulinum toxin and dermal fillers like fat.

Surgical Fee: $5,000 and up; there may be additional fees for the hospital, surgicenter, and anesthesia. The face-lift is the most expensive cosmetic surgical procedure. In large metropolitan areas like Los Angeles and New York, the actual fee for a face-lift operation may range $10-12,000 for the surgeon's fee alone.

Facial Implants

Facial implant surgery is performed to build up various facial features to give the face a more balanced and less flattened appearance. Shape details depend upon the skin and tissues beneath it, including layers of fat, muscle and bone. Implants are placed under the skin to build up contours and areas of over-prominent tissues may be reduced to minimize contour imbalances. Typical regions of contour change include the cheekbones, the jawbone and chin, as well as the lips and the nasolabial creases. More than one region may be treated during one stage. To augment a facial contour, an inert synthetic material is implanted deep below the skin surface and secured with permanent stitches into surrounding tissues so it cannot move around. There are a wide variety of implant materials and shapes and sizes on the market including silicone, Gore-Tex®, elastomer and human tissues. Facial implants are typically fashioned from solid and semi-solid materials, as opposed to gel or saline filled implants that are used in breast augmentation. To reduce a facial contour the underlying tissues are removed by carefully cutting or grinding away excess bone or other tissue.

Surgical Methods

Chin, cheek and jaw augmentation can be performed under local anesthesia, along with intravenous sedation or general anesthesia. You are usually able to leave the hospital or surgicenter after recovery to recuperate at home comfortably.

Cheek Augmentation: Malarplasty is the term for the augmentation or reshaping of the cheeks. In cheek augmentation surgery implants are used to change the underlying structure, which affects the overall balance of facial features. Cheek implants may sometimes be used together with other facial implants, particularly chin implants. In some cases, prominent buccal fat pads in the cheek area may be removed to improve facial contours. This can be done in addition to, or as an alternative to, adding cheek implants. Cheek augmentation involves placing the implant over the cheekbone through an incision made inside the mouth or

Cheek augmentation involves placing the implant over the cheekbone through an incision made inside the mouth or on the outer cheek, or through an opening just beneath the lower eyelash.

on the outer cheek, or through an opening just beneath the lower eyelash. The surgeon creates a pocket in the tissue and then places the implant directly on or below the cheekbone. The incisions are closed with resorbable sutures that dissolve in a week or two. In some cases a small titanium screw may be used to attach the implant to the bone. The implant is inserted through these incisions into a pocket created in the tissue. At the conclusion of the surgery the skin is usually dressed with an elastic strap to reduce swelling.

Chin and Jaw Augmentation: Mentoplasty and Genioplasty are terms used to describe chin surgery that involves the augmentation or reshaping of the chin. Chin augmentation is performed by inserting a silicone implant under the skin. Most often, the incision is made under the chin in the crease and closed with sutures that have to be removed in 5 days. If the incision is inside the mouth it is closed with resorbable sutures that later dissolve. At the end of the surgery the chin is often taped to minimize swelling and a compression strap is worn. Insertion of a jaw implant involves incisions made inside the mouth on either side of the lower lip. The incisions are closed with dissolving stitches.

Chin Reduction: Craniofacial surgery refers to the field of plastic surgery that corrects misshapen jaws caused by misalignment of the teeth and jaws (malocclusion), or mild inadequate tissue development (hypoplasia) which can appear as a recessed upper jaw. Chin reduction surgery involves bone reduction with power bone instruments. If you have a chin deficiency bone surgery or an osteotomy may be necessary where the bone of the chin is moved forward following various oblique bone incisions to reshape the chin. This operation can also be performed in conjunction with nose surgery, as well as liposuction of the face and neck.

Operating Time: 30-90 minutes

Potential Risks or Side Effects

Possible complications include extrusion where the implant works its way back up to the skin's surface, capsular contracture which is a tightening of the scar tissue that can distort the implant, asymmetry and bone erosion. A facial implant can sometimes shift slightly out of alignment, or be placed improperly, and a second operation may be necessary to replace it in its proper position. If an infection occurs the implant may have to be temporarily removed and replaced at a later date. Bone tissue may sometimes become thinner under cheek or chin implants. The treated area may develop numbness that usually resolves after several months, although long-term numbness is a potential complication. In rare cases nerve damage may occur if the implant is resting on one of the facial nerves.

The Recovery Period

After facial implant surgery swelling can be significant and usually peaks 24 to 48 hours afterward. You will be instructed to keep your head elevated, above the level of your heart, when lying down. Swelling and bruising can be minimized by an application of tape or other material for about a week after surgery. Applying cold compresses will reduce swelling and discomfort. The treated area may feel tight and stiff and movement of the mouth may be difficult initially following the surgery. Some difficulty talking, eating and smiling for several days following the surgery is normal. Patients with intra-oral sutures are sometimes placed on a liquid diet for several days until there is enough healing for food particles to come in contact with the stitches. Removable sutures are used for incisions under the chin and are taken out after five to seven days. You can return to work in one to two weeks and resume exercise in three weeks. Avoid contact sports or any activity that may result in the face being jarred or bumped for several weeks. Although most of the significant swelling will subside over several weeks, mild swelling may remain for months until you see your final facial contour changes.

Back to Work: 7-10 days

Alternative Treatment Options

Another way to approach the chin and jaw is with orthodontics, which can treat a malocclusion and misaligned teeth and can significantly change the overall shape of the face. Fat transfer and other filling substances are other methods that can be used to augment cheeks and chins.

Surgical Fee: $2,500-$5,000 depending on the extent of surgery; there may be additional fees for the hospital, surgicenter, and anesthesia.

chapter 16

*Because the nose is the most defining characteristic of the face, a
slight alteration can greatly improve one's appearance.*

Understanding Rhinoplasty—Surgery of the Nose
© 2002 American Academy of Facial
and Reconstructive Plastic Surgery

The Nose

Rhinoplasty can be used to correct a variety of conditions including the
obvious cosmetic issues of how the nose looks and whether it is in proportion with the other facial features, as well as functional problems
including breathing obstructions and traumatic injuries. Breathing problems related to the internal nasal structures can be corrected at the same
time as nose reshaping is performed. When a cosmetic surgeon evaluates
the nose, he or she will study both the frontal view and the profile in addition to the shape and projection of the chin, cheekbones, and upper lip.
Plastic surgeons usually recommend that patients wait until they are at least
age 13 to 15, and possibly older for boys, before undergoing rhinoplasty.
The nose may not be fully developed at a younger age. Assuming you are
in good health, there is no upper age limit for having your nose reshaped.
With age, gravity and the diminishing supportive structures of the nose, the
shape and position of the nose will ultimately change. The nose may
appear longer and the tip eventually droops, thus it is not unusual to have
nasal refinements done at the time of a face-lift procedure or later in life.
A simple elevation of the nasal tip may result in a younger and more attractive appearance. The most common aesthetic complaints regarding the
nose are that: the nose appears too large for your face, there is a bump on
the nasal bridge, the profile is out of proportion, the nose seems too wide
when viewed from the front, the tip droops downward, the tip is too thick,
the nostrils are excessively flared, and the nose is crooked. Previous trauma such as a sports injury or accident may have also contributed to making the nose appear asymmetrical, crooked or enlarged.

The concept of nasal refinement has changed dramatically over the past few decades. In former years, the operation was considered a "reduction rhinoplasty", thereby effectively reducing the size and projection of the nose. Modern rhinoplasty techniques allow the cosmetic surgeon many more options for reshaping the nose. Some noses need to be lengthened, augmented, or narrowed for the best aesthetic result. It is much more possible to have a natural looking nasal correction, instead of the very obvious 'nose job' look of yesteryear. A large portion of the rhinoplasties performed today are revisionary operations to improve a previous surgical result. Instead of erasing all signs of ethnic origins, many patients today prefer to preserve some of the character and ethnic qualities of their original noses while undergoing only subtle refinements. The major limitations in terms of what you can expect as a result of a rhinoplasty procedure have to do with your skin type, skin thickness, the thickness and position of your nasal bones, as well as the skill of the surgeon you select and his or her sense of aesthetics.

Surgical Methods

Rhinoplasty can be performed under general or local anesthesia with intravenous sedation. Incisions are sometimes made inside the rim of the nostrils. In some cases, tiny, inconspicuous incisions are also made on the rim of the nose. Soft tissues of the nose are then separated from the underlying structures and the cartilage and bone causing the deformity are reshaped. The exact nature of that sculpting depends on your particular problem and mission. If the nose is being reduced in size, the nasal bones will be carefully fractured toward the conclusion of the procedure. If your nose needs to be built up in certain areas, grafts using nasal cartilage, ear cartilage, rib cartilage and bone may be used. Other materials can also be used in the nose, including synthetics like silastic implants, human tissue grafts like AlloDerm® or cartilage grafts from a tissue bank. The skin and soft tissues will redrape themselves over the bony architecture of the new nasal shape. Breathing problems may be corrected by a procedure called septoplasty, in which the obstructions are removed, or other methods to improve the airway.

Depending on the technique used, a splint may be placed on the bridge of your nose to hold the tissues in place and to protect your nose. You may also have a small bandage placed under the tip of your nose.

Packing or soft internal splints are sometimes placed inside the nostrils for additional support and to control bleeding. There are two basic ways to perform a rhinoplasty:

Open Technique: The open technique includes an incision across the columella, the small strip of skin that rests between the two nostrils. One major advantage of this technique is the ability to completely visualize the internal structures of the nose and place sutures precisely where they may be required. With this type of rhinoplasty the swelling in the tip may take significantly longer to subside, since some of the tissues have been disrupted. The scar is usually quite small and hidden in the underside of the nose, so it is not very visible. Over time the scar will fade. The stated advantages of this method are that the surgeon is better able to visualize the inner structures of the nose and can sometimes produce a better, more predictable result utilizing a greater variety of surgical techniques.

Closed Technique: The closed technique does not require any external incisions. It usually heals more quickly and does not disturb the tissues as much as the open technique. The surgeon uses instruments that are passed through the nostrils to do the work of resculpting the bones, cartilage and nasal structures. Another type of soft-tissue surgery, alar base reduction, may be used to adjust the width of the nostrils.

Operating Time: 1-3 hours

The Recovery Period

If the nose is being reduced in size, a splint will generally be applied for five to seven days. The nose may be packed lightly with medicated gauze that will require removal in one to two days. In some cases, the nose will be taped with the tip in higher position, which will drop when the tapes and splint are removed. You will be instructed not to get your splint or tape wet. Internal stitches are self-absorbing so they will not require removal. Usually by the end of the first week, splints, bandaging and external sutures will have been removed. There will be some swelling, pressure and stuffiness for several weeks, but you can usually resume light activity after a few days. You will be told to keep your head elevated above the level of your heart for the first few days to reduce swelling. If the nasal bones are fractured, you may have bruising around the eyelid area or bloodshot eyes. Bruising usually peaks at 72 hours and subsides within 10 - 14 days. You may have bleeding from the nose and will be shown how to change your gauze bandages as they get soiled. It will take three weeks before the nose is healed enough to allow full physical activity. You will also need to be careful about blowing your nose. Avoid contact sports or any activity that may risk injury to the nose for four to six weeks. The nose will remain quite tender at this stage. Most eyeglasses will have to be taped to the forehead, off the bridge of the nose, for the first several weeks as the bone sets. It is common to experience acne pustules or oily skin around the nose from the splint. Use broad spectrum sun protection because the skin of the nose may be more prone to burning right after surgery. Your nose may be numb, and the swelling will take longest to settle down in the tip, which can take up to 6-12 months or longer. If your nose has been operated on previously the swelling may take even longer to settle down completely. The thicker your skin the longer it may take to see the final shape in the tip.

If your nose has been operated on previously the swelling may take even longer to settle down completely. The thicker your skin the longer it may take to see the final shape in the tip.

Back to Work: 7-10 days

Potential Risks or Side Effects

Nasal bleeding is common after rhinoplasty. If this becomes excessive, you may be required to return to your doctor's office or the hospital to have your nose repacked or the vessels cauterized. This is not a common occurrence, but more common if you have sneezed inadvertently or bend down after surgery. Infection is also possible but unlikely. There is no such thing as a perfect nose. It is not uncommon for a secondary correction to be required or requested after the nose has settled into its new shape. Some irregularities of cartilage and bone are to be expected and are present in all noses. Secondary nasal surgery will usually not be undertaken for a period of at least 6-12 months until the tissues have fully healed and swelling has resolved.

Alternative Treatment Options

Cosmetic surgeons study your facial features along with your specific concerns to determine whether a complete rhinoplasty or partial rhinoplasty such as a tiplasty, will best accomplish your surgical goals. If your nasal bones are wide or large, it is likely that they will have to be narrowed to achieve a more refined look to the shape of the nose. In some cases, adding a chin implant may achieve the desired look of bringing the facial features into better balance with or without operating on the nose. Nasal implants made of solid silicone rubber or cartilage grafts from septal, ear or rib cartilage are often added to enhance the shape and form of the nose during surgery. In addition, dermal fillers such as fat may be used to fill out subtle defects in the nose, after previous rhinoplasty, injury or in other cases where surgery is not required or requested.

Surgical Fee: $3,500-$8,000 depending on the extent of the procedure; secondary, or revisionary, rhinoplasty fees are usually slightly higher; there may be additional fees for the hospital, surgicenter, and anesthesia. In some cases a deviated septum or history of breathing problems may necessitate nasal surgery. External or cosmetic surgery of the nose in which the shape of the nose is altered is not covered by medical insurance.

"There is certainly no absolute standard of beauty. That precisely is what makes its pursuit so interesting."

John Kenneth Galbraith

Ear Surgery

Ear surgery, or otoplasty, is usually performed to set prominent ears back closer to the head or to reduce the size of one or both ears that are too large in proportion to the size and shape of the face. Ears are considered to be almost fully developed by the age of five. The operation is most commonly performed on children between the ages of five and fourteen. In some cases the surgery is done early so the child avoids teasing and ridicule from other children. Ear surgery is also performed on adults; however, the firmer cartilage of fully developed ears does not have the same capacity for reshaping as in children. Having the procedure at a young age is more desirable because the cartilage is extremely pliable making the surgery easier to perform effectively. Besides protruding ears there are a variety of other ear problems that can be improved surgically. Surgeons can reconstruct ears for those who were born without fully developed ears or who have lost part of the ear due to injury or trauma. Surgery can also be undertaken to improve large or stretched earlobes, or lobes that have large creases due to aging or years of wearing heavy earrings. It is very common to have an earlobe repair or earlobe reduction done in conjunction with face-lift surgery.

COMMON EAR CONDITIONS
- Lop ear: when the tip seems to fold down and forward.
- Cupped ear: usually a very small ear.
- Shell ear: when the curve in the outer rim, as well as the natural folds and creases, are missing.

Surgical Methods

Ear surgery is usually performed as an outpatient procedure under general or local anesthesia with sedation. The surgical technique recommended will depend on the specific problem that needs attention and the cause. One of the most common techniques involves making a small incision in the back of the ear to expose the ear cartilage. The cartilage is then sculpted and bent back towards the head. The surgeon makes a small incision in the back of the ear to expose the ear cartilage and sculpt it into the desired shape. Cartilage is then removed to provide a more natural-looking fold when the procedure is complete. Once the cartilage has been molded, it is then bent back towards the head. Sutures are put in to anchor the ears until healing occurs. The surgeon may put in non-removable stitches to help keep the ears' new shape. Another technique involves a similar incision in the back of the ear. Skin is removed and stitches are used to fold the cartilage back on itself to reshape the ear without removing cartilage. Permanent stitches may be used to help maintain the new shape. In some cases the surgeon may remove a larger portion of cartilage to produce a better fold when the surgery is complete. When only one ear appears to protrude, surgery is usually performed on both ears to create a good balance. Even after undergoing an otoplasty, there is no guarantee that your ears will be perfectly symmetrical.

Operating Time: 1-3 hours

The Recovery Period

Both adults and children are usually up and about within a few hours of surgery. Children will often stay overnight in the hospital until the effects of general anesthesia wear off. The head will be wrapped in a bulky bandage immediately following procedure to promote the best molding and healing. Soft dressings put on the ears will stay on for a few days. Within a few days the bulky bandages will be replaced by a lighter head dressing, similar to a headband, that is worn continuously for two weeks after the procedure to hold the ears in the desired position. Stitches are usually removed, or will dissolve on their own, in about a week. Most people have mild to moderate discomfort following surgery. The ears may throb or ache a little for a few days. You will be instructed not to put any pressure on the ears and to be careful sleeping so as not to disturb the dressings. Any activity in which the ear might be bent should be avoided for one month. Children can go back to school after two weeks if they avoid physical activity and sports.

Back to Work: 7-10 days

Potential Risks or Side Effects

Ear surgery will result in a faint scar in the back of the ear that will fade with time. Ideally there will be a thin white scar after the healing process is completed. The scar can be placed in a natural crease behind the ear so it is not very obvious. Most people can wear their hair back or up without incident after surgery. A small percentage of patients may develop a blood clot on the ear. It may dissolve naturally or can be drawn out with a needle. Occasionally patients develop an infection in the cartilage, which can cause scar tissue to form. Infections are usually treated with antibiotics and, in rare cases, surgery may be required to drain the infected area. It is possible to have an asymmetry between the ears, one is higher than the other, or one is closer to the head than the other. In these cases additional surgery may be needed to revise the position of the ears.

Alternative Treatment Options

Although there are various surgical methods to address protruding ears and other ear deformities, there is no alternative to surgery that will accomplish these goals.

Surgical Fee: $3,000-$5,000; there may be additional fees for the hospital, surgicenter and anesthesia. In some cases, especially in young children, reconstructive ear procedures might be considered a correction of a congenital deformity and may therefore be fully or partially covered by your insurance carrier. Prior approval, including documentation for the necessity of surgery and a second opinion, is generally required.

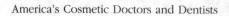

section
III

SURGERY OF THE BODY

Having a beautiful, healthy and active body is something many people desire. Whether your ultimate goal is to look great in your clothes, fit into a smaller size or look better naked, there are a lot of options to consider. For centuries we have been at war with our fat cells, which accounts for the proliferation of diets, miracle pills, power drinks and exercise fads. The fact remains that there are some bodily changes that cannot be significantly altered through diet and exercise alone, although that is the key place to start. In this section you will find an overview of the most common cosmetic surgeries for the body and the breasts, from the least to the most invasive procedure.

chapter 13

"Since the dawn of time, women have looked for secret ways to change their breasts, hoping to trick nature at her own game."

The Breast Book (*Workman Publishing,* 2002)
Maura Spiegel & Lithe Sebesta

The Breasts

In the past few years there has been a surge of breast augmentation procedures worldwide, skyrocketing it to the second most commonly performed cosmetic surgical procedure, next to liposuction, for the past several years in the U.S., according to the American Society for Aesthetic Plastic Surgery. Breast augmentation is performed to increase breast fullness and volume for women with small breasts or those who have experienced a decrease in breast size due to pregnancy or weight loss. There are a wide variety of implant designs, shapes, sizes and textures, all of which have certain advantages and disadvantages. Your surgeon should discuss all the options for breast implants so that you can make an informed decision as to which is best for you.

Breast Augmentation

A breast implant is basically a soft, silicone envelope with various fillers that is surgically implanted under the tissues of your chest to simulate natural breast tissue. The sac may be filled with a gel-like substance or liquid. Although several types of breast implants are available, the model that is used nearly universally for breast augmentation in the US is made of a silicone elastomer shell which is filled with a

COSMETIC BREAST SURGERY
Augmentation: Making them bigger by adding implants
Lift: Making them higher by removing and/or repositioning skin, fat, glandular tissue
Lift with Implants: Making them higher by removing and/or repositioning skin, fat, glandular tissue and adding implants for volume replacement
Reduction: Making them smaller by removing skin, fat, glandular tissue

saline solution. Under certain conditions, including breast reconstruction and secondary procedures, silicone gel implants can be used under approved studies. There are also saline filled adjustable implants that are similar to the standard saline filled implants with the addition of a small connector tube through which the surgeon can adjust the size via injection. This implant requires a second incision to remove the injection port in an additional surgical procedure.

Surgical Methods

A breast augmentation procedure is usually performed in an outpatient surgical center with local anesthesia and intravenous sedation, or general anesthesia. General anesthesia may be chosen for women desiring implant placement below the muscle, since the surgery can be more uncomfortable. The surgery consists of making an incision, lifting the breast tissue, creating a pocket in the chest/breast area, and placing an envelope containing a soft, implant material underneath. An incision may be made in any one of the following places: the crease below the breast, around the areola, under the armpit, or through the navel, which is much less common. The implants can be placed either under the chest muscle or directly under the breasts. Placement considerations include the anatomy of your breasts, breast feeding issues, your lifestyle, and personal preference. Most women have one clear preference. One of the key determining factors is a desire to keep your implants a secret. Having a scar directly on the breast can limit that option, which is why incisions placed in the armpit or in the belly button have become popular.

Operating Time: 1-3 hours

Potential Risks or Side Effects

General complications include nausea, vomiting and fever post anesthesia, hemorrhage, thrombosis or abnormal clotting, and skin necrosis resulting from insufficient blood flow to the skin. Breast implants are classified as mechanical devices by the U.S. Food and Drug Administration. As such, they are not considered lifetime devices. Depending on your age when you have implants placed, you will likely undergo implant removal with or without replacement one or more times during your lifetime. Some women may keep their implants intact for twenty plus years; others will need them exchanged or replaced in six months or some other time frame. It is impossible to predict with any degree of certainty how long your implants will last. Recent scientific reports suggest that implant life is an average of 16 years. Other important safety issues that surround breast implants include implant rupture rates and the incidence of capsular contracture, which can cause painful hardening of the breast or distort its appearance. The concerns regarding breast augmentation include the surgery itself, the implants, and the issue of mammography readings. The risks involved with breast augmentation have received a lot of attention. All

CHOICES IN BREAST IMPLANTS

Filling Substance
- Saline
- Silicone Gel

Incision Placement
- Under the breast-inframammary
- Around the nipple areola complex-perioareolar
- Under the armpit-transaxillary
- Through the navel-transumbilical

Implant Texture
- Coated
- Smooth

Implant Shape
- Round
- Teardrop or anatomical

operations carry some risk and the possibility of the need for a second, or sometimes a third procedure, is especially high with breast augmentation surgery. Another topic of concern is the potential for interference with mammography readings that could possibly delay breast cancer detection. It may be difficult to distinguish calcium deposits formed in the scar tissue from a lesion when interpreting the mammogram. When making an appointment for a mammogram, you will be instructed to inform the radiologist that you have implants, and to make sure that the technician uses special techniques and instrumentation to obtain the best mammogram reading and to avoid rupturing the implant. Women who are considering breast augmentation are also advised to have a baseline mammogram before having surgery, depending on their age at the time of surgery and family history. If you are not happy with your implants, it is possible to have them removed at any time. If you have had the implants in place for several years, depending on the size of the implant and the quality of your breast tissue, removing them may result in a droopier breast shape. In this case a breast lift procedure may be recommended.

The Recovery Period

You will need someone to drive you home, and you will need assistance at home over the next couple of days. Your breasts will be wrapped with gauze bandage and you will need a surgical bra or elastic band for additional protection and support. You will be instructed to keep your dressings dry. You also may have drainage tubes placed in the incision for several days to help eliminate excess fluid. After five to seven days the gauze dressing will be removed and you may be required to wear a non-under wired support or sports bra continuously for several weeks. Your breasts will be taped in place under the bra and will appear firm, swollen and sitting high on your chest at first. As the swelling resolves, the breast implants will drop into a more normal position and shape. You will be told to minimize arm movements and to bend from the knees only as needed. Elbows should not be raised higher than the level of your armpits. You will heal more quickly if you avoid stretching and lifting to avoid separating the muscle and tissue surrounding the implants. You may be able to resume work within a week or two after surgery. You should continue to avoid aerobic activity for three to four weeks until the soreness has subsided. The stitches will come out within a week to ten days and swelling will gradually subside over several weeks. The scars will remain pink for several months and should be kept out of direct sunlight.

Back to Work: 7-10 days

BREAST IMPLANT RISKS

This is only a partial list of some of the most common risks associated with breast implants

- Rippling, indentations, palpability
- Implant rupture or leakage
- Capsular contracture or hardening of the breast due to scar tissue
- Leak, rupture or implant deflation
- Temporary or permanent loss of sensation in the nipple or breast tissue
- Formation of calcium deposits in surrounding tissue causing pain and hardening
- Implant shifting

Alternative Treatment Options

New implant filling substances continue to be under development. At the present time a thicker silicone gel is available outside of the U.S. that is considered less likely to rupture due to the texture and consistency of the gel filler. It is possible that this implant may be available in the U.S. in the next several years. A hyaluronic acid gel filler developed in Sweden to be injected into breast tissues is currently being investigated as a possible alternative to breast implants, but it is estimated to be several years away. Fat injections directly into the breast are not recommended as an alternative to breast implantation due to the possible interference with mammography readings.

Surgical Fee: $3,000-$7,000 plus the price of the implants

Breast Lift

A breast lift, or mastopexy, is a surgical procedure to raise and reshape breasts that have sagged as a result of pregnancy, nursing and the natural force of gravity. It can also reduce the size of the areola, the darker skin surrounding the nipple. Shape and balance come into play and there is no set formula for every woman. A breast lift can also be combined with the placement of an implant in some cases where volume needs to be enhanced or replaced.

Surgical Methods

Several different techniques can be used to correct this condition, depending on the degree of sagging. Surgery consists of removing excess skin from around the areola, and possibly from the bottom of the breast, with shifting of the skin of the breast to tighten the skin envelope, also insertion of additional volume, such as an implant for added projection and smoothing of the skin can be added. This elevates the position of the nipple and areola to a more youthful position. Specific breast lift techniques vary, but they generally fall into the more traditional incision pattern and the modified or scar-saving techniques. The most common technique is the traditional anchor incision, also called the inverted T or Wise pattern, which involves a scar around the nipple areola complex, a vertical extension and horizontally under the breast. This technique is also commonly used in breast reductions. In general, the more tissue that is removed, the more shaping is possible. In women with extensive sagging from multiple childbirths, breast feeding, age and weight fluctuations, the skin may be so stretched and thinned that a smaller incision will not allow the surgeon to remove sufficient tissue to lift the breast. In these cases, longer incisions may be required. The vertical mastopexy falls somewhere in-between the traditional and minimal scar technique, and is widely suitable for many types of breasts. The periareolar mastopexy, which involves an incision placed only around the areola, is usually reserved for women with small breasts that are only mildly droopy where very little skin needs to be removed.

The procedure is usually performed in an outpatient surgical center. Breast lift surgery can be performed under local anesthesia with intravenous sedation, or under general anesthesia. The standard breast lift has four components; the areola is reduced, breast tissue is repositioned, the nipple and areola are elevated to a better position, and excess skin and breast tissue is removed so that a new skin envelope is formed. The most common procedure still involves an anchor-shaped incision following the natural contour of the breast. The incision outlines the area from which breast skin will be removed and defines the new location for the nipple. When the excess skin has been removed, the nipple and areola are moved to the higher position. The skin surrounding the areola is then brought down and together to reshape the breast. Stitches are usually located around the areola, in a vertical line extending downward from the nipple area, with or without a suture line along the lower crease of the breast, depending on the method used.

Operating Time: 1-3 hours

BREAST LIFT TECHNIQUES

One Scar: Periareolar Incision, just around the nipple, also called "doughnut" or "concentric"

Two Scars: Vertical Incision, around the nipple with a vertical extension, also called "lollipop"

Three Scars: Anchor Incision, also called "Wise Pattern", around the nipple with a vertical extension and an incision partially or all the way under the breast horizontally

The Recovery Period

An elastic bandage or a surgical bra over gauze dressings must be worn after surgery. The breasts will be bruised, swollen and uncomfortable for several days. Within a few days, a soft support bra will replace the bandages or surgical bra. This bra must be worn constantly for several weeks over a layer of gauze. The stitches will be removed after a week or two. You will be instructed to wear a bra for support for several weeks to months. Underwire bras may cause a blister on the delicate postoperative tissues. You may be up and about in a day or two, but you should avoid lifting anything over your head or engage in strenuous sports for three to four weeks. You may be instructed to avoid sexual activity for a week or longer. Breast skin can be very dry following surgery and careful application of moisturizer several times a day can alleviate itching. Some loss of feeling in your nipples and breast skin caused by postoperative swelling can occur. Sensation usually returns as the swelling subsides over the following four to six weeks. In some cases it may last a year or more and occasionally may be permanent.

Back to Work: 7-10 days

Potential Risks or Side Effects

Bleeding and infection following a breast lift are uncommon, but can cause scars to widen. It is possible to have unevenly positioned nipples, permanent loss of sensation around the nipples and breast asymmetry. Perhaps the most common risks are the quality of healing and your acceptance of the resulting scars. A breast lift will result in permanent visible scars, especially if you are prone to scarring problems such as keloids. They can remain lumpy and red for months and then gradually become less obvious, ideally eventually fading to thin white lines. With a breast lift the most significant trade off for better-positioned breasts is the appearance and permanence of scars that may take months to one year before they flatten out and the pigment fades. The operation usually does not affect your ability to breastfeed, since your milk ducts and nipples are left intact. If the ability to breastfeed is an important consideration for you, make sure this is reviewed in detail with your surgeon before going ahead with surgery.

Alternative Treatment Options

A breast augmentation can also help lift the breast by increasing volume, but is not really considered an alternative to a breast lift. If your skin envelope has been stretched, having a larger implant placed may result in increasing sag. The best results are usually achieved in women with small, sagging breasts. Breasts of any size can be lifted, but the results may not last as well in very large, heavy breasts where some tissue may need to be removed to result in a more pleasing shape and appearance. The results of a breast lift will not keep the breasts firm forever. The effects of gravity, pregnancy, aging and weight fluctuations will eventually take their toll again. A mastopexy may need to be repeated in ten or more years.

> *A breast augmentation can also help lift the breast by increasing volume, but is not really considered an alternative to a breast lift.*

Surgical Fee: $4,000-$7,000; there may be additional fees for the hospital, surgicenter and anesthesia.

Breast Reduction

The motivation for having a breast reduction varies considerably with age. For teenagers and younger women it is primarily an emotional decision. As women get older it becomes more of a practical choice. The decision is as much social and emotional as it is physical. Breast reduction is a procedure in which excess tissue is removed to make the breast smaller and less heavy. Women who consider this procedure are those who suffer from back and neck pain, grooves in the shoulders from bra straps pain in the breasts, and rashes that are caused by heavy breasts. Sometimes heavy breasts can even exacerbate an existing condition like arthritis. Some women are bothered by the psychological embarrassment of large breasts, or uneven breasts, or have trouble finding clothes or bras that fit. For women who are more physically active, big breasts can be a real limitation to jogging, aerobics and swimming. Bouncing can also hurt and cause necks to snap. Women rarely choose breast reduction surgery only to change the way they look. They have it done because the size of their breasts is affecting their comfort and health. These procedures aren't just about having a new look; they represent a means to an end to the physical symptoms and discomfort that some women have suffered with for years, and sometimes decades. If you are more than 30 pounds, or twenty percent, over your ideal weight, some surgeons will recommend that you lose the weight before surgery. Weight loss after the breast reduction may result in additional unpredictable loss of volume and this could be accompanied by sagging.

Surgical Methods

The procedure is usually performed in an outpatient surgical center or a hospital facility. If you are having more than one procedure overnight hospitalization may be recommended. Although most often performed under general anesthesia, breast reduction can also be performed under local anesthesia with intravenous sedation. Most often the incisions for breast reduction are similar to those used for the breast lift technique. Breast reduction surgery is a trade-off between the extent of the scars and the extent of the shaping of the new breast and of the size reduction possible. The most common technique involves an anchor-shaped incision that circles the areola, extends downward and follows the natural curve of the crease beneath the breast. Incisions outline the area of skin, breast tissue and fat to be removed, and also outline the new position for the nipple. In most cases, the nipples remain attached to their blood vessels and nerves. Excess glandular tissue, fat, and skin are removed, and the nipple and areola are moved into their new position. The surgeon then brings the skin from both sides of the breast down and around the areola, shaping the new contour of the breast. If the breasts are very large or pendulous, the nipples and areola may have to be completely removed and grafted into a higher position. The surgeon removes excess glandular tissue, fat and skin, and moves the nipple and areola into their new position. Skin that was formerly located above the nipple is brought down and joined to reshape the breast. Sutures are used to close the incisions, giving the breast its new contour. Stitches are usually located around the areola, in a vertical line extending downward, and along the lower crease of the breast. The resulting scars around the areola, below it, and in the crease under the breast, are permanent. In general, the more skin that is removed, the better shape you can expect. If you have a history of keloid scarring, it may be wise to investigate modified scar breast reduction techniques to eliminate some of the scarring involved. Skin quality and skin elasticity are the key determining factors.

Some Common Breast Reduction Incisions and Their Indications

Free Nipple Graft: In women with large, pendulous breasts and thin, stretched skin may need a nipple graft technique. Because the nipple is so far from where the surgeon wants to place it, the nipple and areola are removed from the breast and grafted back onto the reduced breast. This procedure involves an anchor-shaped incision that circles the areola, extends downward, and follows the natural curve of the crease beneath the breast. While some women recover breast sensation after nipple grafting, doctors usually advise patients that it is not always possible. Most patients who undergo a free nipple graft are not able to breast-feed after surgery.

Pedicle Methods: The most common methods for breast reduction involve a pedicle, or platform, of tissue that is not excised so that nerve loss or areola necrosis is minimized. There are numerous variations of this technique that may be recommended, depending on the size of your breasts. Pedicle techniques are recommended for moderately large or heavy breasts. The surgeon removes excess breast tissue and skin while preserving a central breast mound. The nipple and areola are repositioned but remain attached to their blood and nerve supplies. The incisions are usually made under the crease of the breast, sometimes extending out

> *Although the ideal candidate for this technique has moderately large breasts and elastic skin, many experienced surgeons apply modified scar techniques to all breast types.*

to beneath the arm, around the nipple and areola, and vertically down from the nipple. In many cases nipple sensation is preserved, although you should be prepared for some loss of sensation. Between 40 and 60 percent of women are unable to breastfeed after this surgery.

Short Scar Techniques: There are a variety of short scar techniques that aim to abolish the medial scar under the breast fold. In some cases, techniques can be used that eliminate the long vertical part of the scar. In most cases, the nipples remain attached to their blood vessels and nerves. Reduction of the breast with the vertical technique eliminates the infra-mammary scar. Although the ideal candidate for this technique has moderately large breasts and elastic skin, many experienced surgeons apply modified scar techniques to all breast types.

Liposuction-Only Breast Reduction: When only fatty tissue needs to be removed, liposuction alone can be used to reduce breast size. As you get older, breasts are made up of more fat than gland. Liposuction, a procedure in which excess fatty tissue is removed from a specific area of the body by means of a suction device, is sometimes used to remove excess fat from the armpit area, although some surgeons also use this procedure to remove excess fatty tissue from the breast. Instead of a large skin incision, liposuction involves a few small punctures to remove excess fatty tissue from the breast.

Operating Time: 2-5 hours

The Recovery Period

After surgery your breasts will be wrapped in an elastic bandage or a surgical bra over gauze dressings. You may have small drainage tubes coming out of the incisions to help drain some of the excess fluid for a period of three to five days or longer as needed. The bandages will be removed a day or two after surgery, though you will continue to wear the surgical bra around the clock for several weeks. In most cases, stitches will be removed in 7-14 days. Sometimes dissolvable sutures may be used. You will have some pain and tenderness for the first week, especially when you move around or cough. A small amount of fluid draining from the incision, and crusting, is normal. Random, shooting pains may be experienced for a few months. Some loss of sensation can be expected in your nipples and breast skin, caused by swelling that usually fades over the next six weeks. In some cases it may last a year or more, and occasionally it may be permanent. Although you may be up and about in a few days, avoid lifting or pushing anything heavy for three or four weeks, and try to rest as much as possible for the first month post-op. Most women can return to work and social activities in about two weeks, but you should plan on limiting exercise until your energy level returns to normal. You will be instructed to avoid any activity that will elevate your heart rate for the first 10 days. Sexual arousal can cause your incisions to swell and possible bleeding. Refrain from anything but gentle contact with your breasts for about six weeks. If breast skin is very dry following surgery, moisturizer can be applied several times a day, but the suture area must be kept dry at all times. The first menstruation following surgery may cause breasts to swell and hurt. Although much of the swelling and bruising will disappear in the first few weeks, it may be six months before the breasts settle into their final new shape. The shape may fluctuate in response to your hormonal shifts, weight changes, and pregnancy.

Back to Work: 7-10 days

Potential Risks or Side Effects

Breast reduction scars are extensive and permanent. They often remain lumpy and red for months, and then gradually become less obvious, sometimes eventually fading to thin white lines. Scars can often be placed inconspicuously enough so that you can even wear low-cut tops. Another potential complication that is more common with free nipple graft methods is the loss of pigment around the areola. This can be improved if necessary with micro pigmentation or tattooing. The procedure can also leave slightly mismatched breasts or unevenly positioned nipples. Some patients develop small sores around their nipples after surgery that can be easily treated with antibiotic creams. Future breastfeeding may not be possible, since the surgery removes many of the milk ducts leading to the nipples. In rare cases, there may be a permanent loss of sensation. It is rare but possible that the nipple and areola may lose their blood supply and the tissue will suffer from necrosis and have to be treated while it heals.

Alternative Treatment Options

An alternative to breast reduction could be a breast lift. While this procedure can raise and reshape breasts that have sagged as a result of pregnancy, nursing and the natural force of gravity, and can reduce the size of the areola, it does not significantly reduce the overall size and weight of the breast. Liposuction may be also be used in breast reduction, especially in younger patients with firm skin and very fatty breast composition.

Surgical Fee: $5,000-$9,000; there may be additional fees for the hospital, surgicenter and anesthesia. In some cases, insurance coverage may be obtainable depending on the criteria of your individual carrier.

chapter 19

Males made up 15 percent of all cosmetic plastic surgery patients in 2002, with 966,821 patients.

American Society of Plastic Surgeons

PECTORAL IMPLANTS

For men born with a congenital defect or who have suffered an injury, implants may be used to enlarge the bulk and projection of the pectoral muscles. Increasing the definition of your pectoralis muscles can only be accomplished through exercise. Pectoral implants will not improve your chest contours in such a way that you will be able to see a clear distinct edge of the muscle.

Surgical Methods

Surgery is performed under general anesthesia or intravenous sedation. Your surgeon may also perform the procedure with the aid of an endo-scope. A small incision is made in the armpit and a cavity is created under the pectoralis muscle. The muscle is not divided from its attachments to the rib cage or breast bone. A solid silastic implant is placed directly beneath your pectoral muscle. The surgeon makes a small incision in the armpit then inserts the implant endoscopically using a thin tube with a very small camera on the end in order to guide the physician with a great amount of precision. Following the path of the incision, the surgeon places the implants under the pectoral muscle. The incisions are then sutured and the surgery is complete. The implants are held in place by the overlying chest muscle or by sutures that are temporarily visible through the skin.

The Recovery Period

In most cases, patients are able to go home the day of surgery. You can expect to be considerably sore for the first few days to one week. Your dressing and sutures will be removed in a few days. Some surgeons do not apply incision dressings or drains after the surgery. In these cases, patients do not need to worry about changing bandages etc. You will be instructed to wear an elastic bandage or vest to reduce swelling. Unlike female breast implant surgery, pectoral implants do not carry the risk of leaking or rupture. The silicone implant used for men is soft but solid, unlike the typical fluid-filled breast implants used in women.

Back to Work 7-10 days

Potential Risks or Side Effects

The risks are similar to those of breast enlargement in women, except that there is no risk of deflation since the implants are not filled. If your implants are placed too lateral (near the arm) or too high (near the collar bone), surgery may be required to reposition them. Displacement of chest implants is also a possible complication. If the implant moves or is not held in place correctly by the pectoral muscle, further surgery may be required. In extreme cases, the implant may need to be removed permanently. If you develop an infection, it normally will be treated with antibiotics and/or implant removal. Seromas may develop immediately after surgery that may persist and require evacuation with a needle or surgery. Numbness of the inner upper arm may occur as a result of the nerve becoming disrupted, stretched, or cauterized during surgery. The numbness usually will resolve within the first few months. If you have a complication from your chest implants and decide that you want them removed, it can be performed through the same incision, and recovery is faster than from the original surgery.

Alternative Treatment Options

Although there are no other procedures that will substantially enlarge the chest, exercise, especially weight lifting, should always be considered an alternative method.

Surgical Fee: $4,000 – $6,000 plus the cost of the implants, hospital or surgicenter and anesthesia.

chapter 20

More than 14,000 men underwent gynecomastia surgery last year,
ranking the procedure sixth amongst men having cosmetic surgery.

American Society of Plastic Surgeons © 2003

GYNECOMASTIA

Gynecomastia by is a condition that affects men's breasts making them appear enlarged due to an excess of skin, fat and gland. The word literally translates as "women-like breasts." This procedure surgically corrects the problem by removing fat and/or glandular tissue from a man's chest. The result is a flatter, firmer, more aesthetically pleasing contoured chest. If you're a man who has enlarged breasts, you probably have a long list of personal benefits that a breast reduction procedure would offer you. Male breast reduction can eliminate the look of having enlarged, fatty breasts and create a flatter, firmer chest with a better contour to the chest area. This procedure may be discouraged if you are very overweight. The use of anabolic steroids, estrogen-containing medications, marijuana use and impaired liver function may contribute to gynecomastia. Your surgeon may also recommend a mammogram to rule out the possibility of breast cancer. The mammogram will also help the surgeon determine the best surgical procedure based on how much fat and glandular tissue is contained within the breasts

Surgical Methods

Gynecomastia reduction is most often performed on an outpatient basis. There are two different approaches to male breast reduction, but they are frequently combined. It will depend on whether the condition is caused by excess glandular tissue or excess fatty tissue. If excess glandular tissue is the primary cause of enlarged male breasts, the tissue will be cut out with a scalpel. This may be done alone or in conjunction with liposuction. Typically, an incision is made on the edge of the areola. Working through the incision, the surgeon removes excess glandular tissue and fat. If excess fatty tissue is the primary cause of enlarged male breasts, the procedure is slightly different. In this case, the excess fatty tissue will be removed by liposuction. A small incision, less than a half-inch in length, is made around the edge of the areola. The incision also may be placed under the arm. A cannula is attached to a vacuum pump then inserted into the incision. The surgeon moves the cannula through the layers beneath the skin, breaking up the fat and suctioning it out. In cases where large amounts of fat or glandular tissue have been removed, skin may not shrink sufficiently to the new smaller breast contour and excess skin may have to be removed. These incisions may be placed around the areola, straight down the front of the breast and in the crease under the breast. This procedure is typically reserved for men who have a massive weight loss resulting in excess skin. A small drain may be inserted through a separate incision to draw off excess fluids. The incisions usually are covered with a dressing and the chest may be wrapped to keep the skin firmly in place.

> *A small incision, less than a half-inch in length, is made around the edge of the areola. The incision also may be placed under the arm.*

Operating Time: 1-3 hours

The Recovery Period

For the first few days, you can expect to feel uncomfortable, swollen and bruised. To reduce swelling, an elastic pressure garment may be worn for a week or two continuously and for a few weeks longer at night. You will be encouraged to walk around on the day of procedure. Stitches generally will be taken out five to six days following the procedure or they may be resorbable. Your surgeon may advise you to avoid sexual activity and heavy exercise for about three weeks. You also will be instructed to refrain from any sport or job function that risks a blow to the chest area for at least four weeks. It may take up to three months or more before the final results of your procedure are apparent. You also should avoid exposing the scars to the sun for at least six weeks as they are healing. Sunlight can permanently affect the skin's pigmentation, causing the scar to darken.

Back to Work: 4-7 days

Potential Risks and Complications

Specific risks include visible or raised scars, permanent pigment changes in the breast area and slightly mismatched breasts or nipples. A second procedure may be performed to remove additional tissue or smooth out rippling if necessary. Temporary side effects include loss of breast sensation or numbness, which may last up to a year. Removing the gland can sometimes result in a hollow or divot of the chest wall. More extensive procedures will also leave larger scars, but the scars from just liposuction are usually quite small and hidden.

Alternative Treatment Options

Surgical alternatives are liposuction or liposuction with skin excision, which is rarely used at this time. There are no effective non-surgical alternatives for reducing gynecomastia. Weight loss can help conceal the condition, but enlarged breast tissue may still remain even after substantial weight reduction.

Surgical Fee: $2,500-$5,000; there may be additional fees for the hospital, surgicenter, and anesthesia

"Good looks are a woman's most fungible asset, exchangeable for social position, money, even love. But, dependent on a body that ages, it is an asset that a woman uses or loses."

The Beauty Business: Pots of Promise
The Economist, May 24, 2003

LIPOSUCTION

Fat cells play numerous metabolic roles in the body including as an energy source, a storage place, interaction with insulin and hormone synthesis, to name a few. Adult fat cells are thought to be incapable of multiplying. There are a fixed number distributed in a genetically predetermined fashion throughout the body. Regardless of the function, as you gain weight these cells expand. As you lose weight, they contract but the number and distribution remain essentially unchanged, which accounts for why thin people may still complain about localized fatty deposits that don't go away, even at their ideal weight. Dieting reduces your weight and overall size. Liposuction reduces the overall number of fat cells and affects shape and contour so future weight gain or loss won't be noticed as much in the areas that were treated as in non-treated areas. It is a safe and effective way to remove unsightly bulges from almost any area to produce an improved shape and contour. This is why liposuction has consistently been the most popular cosmetic surgical procedure in the world for the past several years. Liposuction has come a long way since its introduction in the mid 1970s and modern techniques have made it safer and simpler for both surgeons and patients.

Fat deposits that don't respond to the usual litany of exercise and diet regimens are ideal targets for liposuction. If you are overweight only in certain areas of your body, for example saddlebags, you would have to lose a larger amount of weight in order to shrink the size of your thighs. The weight will come off everywhere including the breasts and face, and not just where you need it most. Most body parts can be suctioned for better contour and reduced volume, from the face down to the ankles. The most popular areas for women are the abdomen, inner thighs, outer thighs, hips, flanks and knees. Liposuction can even be used to reduce heavy breasts in some women. The trend is to treat areas of the body "circumferentially," instead of removing fat deposits from selected spots.

The trend is to treat areas of the body "circumferentially," instead of removing fat deposits from selected spots.

Sections like the abdomen, hips, waist, and all around the thighs and knees, and upper arms can be combined to maximize the potential for the skin to shrink after the fat is removed. You should evaluate your body in distinct units, like the upper abdomen, lower abdomen, knees, and prioritize the areas that would benefit most from recontouring. Before having liposuction, your cosmetic surgeon should discuss your lifestyle, shape and body weight fluctuations. If you have a history of an eating disorder like bulimia, anorexia, binge eating, or have been on prescription weight control medications, tell your surgeon in advance. Patients who are very overweight may have to undergo these procedures in stages. Patients who exceed their ideal weight by 50% or more will be told to lose weight prior to undergoing a liposuction procedure.

Surgical Methods

Advances in liposuction techniques have greatly improved the results you can achieve. The procedure is very straightforward. Tiny incisions of approximately one quarter inch long are made at the sites where fat is to be removed and a wetting solution is infused to provide anesthesia, reduce bleeding and improve fat extraction. This requires careful monitoring to avoid toxicity and must be performed by those experienced with local anesthesia. The surgeon uses various sizes and dimensions of 'cannula,' hollow, tubular instruments with holes at one end, to trap the fat. The cannula is attached to suction tubing through which the excess fat is evacuated. These instruments come in various shapes, lengths and sizes depending on the thickness and location of the fat. They have highly polished surfaces to slip through the fatty tissues with minimum friction or damage, and are frequently blunt-tipped to prevent cutting through the skin. Cannulae are inserted under the skin moved in a back and forth and crisscross fashion within the fat, essentially pushing it aside while protecting the vessels and nerves. Fat is suctioned out through one or several holes at the tip, measured, and the patient is checked for symmetry. The procedure is completed when a safe level of fat removal and the desired contour has been achieved. The patient is then monitored closely to make sure that enough fluid hydration has been received.

Tumescent: "Tumescent" anesthesia has had perhaps the most significant impact of all developments in liposuction. Warmed tumescent liquid, a diluted solution containing Lidocaine, epinephrine and intravenous fluid, is injected into the area to be treated. As the liquid enters the fat, it becomes swollen, firm and blanched. The "wet" technique, and the "super-wet" technique, referring to the amount of fluids injected, are variations of the tumescent technique. The expanded fat compartments allow the liposuction cannula to travel smoothly beneath the skin as the fat is removed. The saline softens the fat, the adrenaline decreases the blood loss and bruising, and the anesthesia provides relief from discomfort. For small amounts of fat, the tumescent solution may be the only anesthetic given or it can be supplemented with sedatives to put you in a sleepy state. General anesthesia may also be used for longer procedures involving multiple areas.

Ultrasound: Ultrasonic sound waves, like shock waves, are transmitted into the fatty tissues from the tip of the cannula probe. The fat cells are melted or liquefied and then removed by low-pressure vacuum through a suction tube. Ultrasonic liposuction is often reserved for large volumes and multiple areas, and more difficult areas to contour where the deep fat is thicker, and thus harder to extract; i.e. back rolls, upper abdomen, and flanks. It is usually combined with traditional liposuction when both the deeper fat and more superficial fat are being removed. When previous liposuction has been done, it may be useful to soften the scar tissue that develops to make it easier for the surgeon to get the fat out. External ultrasound waves can also be used with liposuction in lower frequencies to soften fat deposits from the skin's surface.

Power Assisted Lipoplasty: One of the latest advances in technology for liposuction is the addition of power. The cannulae used are motor-driven so they vibrate which makes removing fat easier and faster for the surgeon. The primary advantage is that there is less physical exertion required for the surgeon to remove the fat with this method.

VASER® Assisted Lipoplasty: The VASER® system utilizes probes with a grooved design and continuous bursts of ultrasonic vibrational energy to selectively target larger fat cells which are then removed by suction.

Liposculpture: Liposculpture is a term for the removal of small to medium amounts of fat in rather normal to full areas to sharpen features, accentuate the muscles beneath and create a more cut appearance in the neck, lower cheeks, upper abdomen, outer buttocks, calves and ankles.

Operating Time: 1-4 hours

The Recovery Period

Most people have liposuction on an outpatient basis and go home the same day. For large volume procedures, or multiple sites, it may be recommended that you stay overnight in the hospital or clinic. During the two days following the procedure, you can expect significant swelling, but this rapidly subsides within days and resolves quickly over the next three weeks. You will weigh more right after liposuction than before surgery. Your face, feet and hands may swell up from all the fluids pumped into you. Swelling travels down like everything else, so don't be surprised if you're puffy and bruised in places you didn't have suctioned. There will also be numbness in some areas. Showering is usually permitted after two days. Most surgeons will request that you continue to wear a compression garment for several weeks after surgery. Many people can return to work or limited activity within two to four days, and resume an exercise program as tolerated in 10–14 days. Use a lubricant like petrolatum to keep incisions soft and stop scabs from forming. You may find yourself itching after surgery. Use a rich moisturizer, a loofah in the shower, and take warm oatmeal baths to help soothe dry skin. You can see your new shape best after three weeks, when most of the swelling has subsided. Residual swelling settles gradually over the next three to six months.

Back to Work: 3-10 days, depending on the extent of the procedure

Potential Risks or Side Effects

A major benefit of liposuction surgery is that the scars needed are tiny. Small slit-like scars can be placed in hidden areas like in the belly button, in the crease under the buttocks, and inside the knee, so they are well concealed. These scars generally heal well and they are rarely a problem. After surgery a compression garment will be placed. Wearing the girdle for a few weeks will hold everything in and keep swelling to a minimum. Most patients actually feel better with some support and compression. The risks from liposuction are most often related to the expertise of the surgeon as well as the anesthesiologist. Specific risks from the tumescent technique include rare complications like pulmonary edema, which is a collection of fluid in the lungs that may occur if too much fluid is administered. Lidocaine toxicity which can occur if there is too much Lidocaine in the solution, is another potential deadly complication. If the surgeon injects too much of the solution, overworking the heart or drowning in fluids are possible consequences. Anti-embolism boots are often used during surgery to prevent a blood clot from forming in the deep veins of the pelvis or legs. A fat embolus can also occur where a bit of fat travels into the bloodstream. The risk of a seroma is possible, especially after ultrasound techniques, and more common in areas like the abdomen and chest. In these cases, the surgeon may drain the excess fluid to relieve pressure. Generally, the greater the volume of fat and fluids removed, the greater the risks. In some cases, a touch-up may be done six months after the initial procedure to refine an area that has previously been treated. If you have had liposuction and the skin is loose, additional liposuction will only make the skin look worse. A skin excision procedure may be recommended instead. The results of liposuction are permanent, as long as you keep your weight stable. If you gain weight after liposuction, you will tend to gain it back in the areas not suc-

BODY AREAS THAT CAN BE LIPOSUCTIONED

- Chin, neck, jowls
- Cheeks
- Upper Arms
- Forearms
- Posterior and Anterior Axillary folds
- Breasts
- Upper and Lower Abdomen
- Waist
- Upper Back and Back Rolls
- Upper hips and flanks
- Banana Rolls
- Outer Thighs
- Inner Thighs
- Anterior and Posterior Thighs
- Inner Knees
- Calves
- Ankles

tioned since the normal number of fat cells are still there and will continue to expand. There are still fat cells in the areas that were suctioned. If you do gain fat in other areas of the body that weren't your primary trouble spots, it is usually very responsive to diet and exercise.

Alternative Treatment Options

The ideal patient for liposuction is at or close to a normal weight. Some doctors will perform liposuction on patients who are thirty pounds or more overweight, or over 30% of their ideal body weight. The best pre-liposuction weight is one you can maintain without starving yourself. It is better to lose some weight before surgery and more afterwards. If you put on a few pounds after liposuction, you will lose some of the benefit of your result. If you lose some weight

Basically, 5,000 cc's of fat and fluids is the maximum amount that is considered safe to remove at one stage, depending on your size

after, your result will look that much better. Every patient complains to her cosmetic surgeon after liposuction, "couldn't you have taken a little more fat out?" It is not uncommon to undergo a small touch-up procedure six months later. There are limits, based on your size, weight, overall health and tolerance for surgery. Basically, 5,000 cc's of fat and fluids is the maximum amount that is considered safe to remove at one stage, depending on your size at the start. Anything over that amount is considered 'large volume liposuction' and can be more risky. If you have several areas you want suctioned, you can easily get up to that level rather quickly. The choices are to lose weight before having liposuction, or have it done in multiple stages. Although liposuction is an effective method for removing fat deposits, it does not cure cellulite, tighten loose skin, or affect the fat that lies underneath the muscle layer. When the degree of skin elasticity is not easy to assess, a staged procedure may be a good solution. The liposuction is done first, and if not enough skin contracts, skin excision and internal tightening can be done at a later stage. Fat from other body parts can be suctioned out and injected back to smooth and fill out dents and add curves. Liposuction can be used to delicately recontour legs from the ankles, calves, and knees up to the inner and outer thighs, taking inches off the circumference of the leg. Calves and anterior thighs are tricky because they are often largely muscle, but suctioning even small amounts can make a big difference in the overall shape. Liposuction of the legs may take longer than other areas to fully settle down, because swelling tends to travel downward and rest below the knee. This procedure is usually best left for colder months when you can easily cover up bruising and swelling under clothing.

The more elastic the skin, the better liposuction works. If you have flabby skin due to pregnancies, aging or weight fluctuations, liposuction can potentially make it look worse. Some areas of fat deposits are less forgiving than others and more often lead to sagging skin; for example, upper arms, inner thighs, knees, abdomen and the neck. If your ultimate goal is to be taut, a tummy tuck, thigh lift, or lower body lift, which involve tightening underlying muscles and removing and redraping excess skin, are the only viable options. The trade-off is that the scars are significant and the recovery period is considerably longer than with liposuction alone.

Surgical Fee: Liposuction can range from $2,500 for one small area to $8-$10,000 for several areas done at one stage. The number of incisions made as well as the amount of fat removed contributes to the fees.

chapter 22

"A great body is your best body, at whatever age."

Ageless Beauty (Hyperion, 1998)
by Dayle Haddon

ABDOMINOPLASTY

Abdominoplasty, commonly known as a "tummy tuck," is performed to remove excess skin and fat from the middle and lower abdomen and to tighten the muscles of the abdominal wall. The best candidates are in relatively good shape with fat deposits with loose abdominal skin that does not respond to diet or exercise. If there is a large fat accumulation, liposuction may be suggested first to remove excess fatty deposits, followed by an abdominoplasty to address loose skin and muscles at a second stage. If you have scarring from previous abdominal surgery, your doctor may recommend against abdominoplasty.

Women whose abdominal muscles and skin have been stretched out from multiple pregnancies, as well as older women who have a loss of skin elasticity due to age or weight fluctuations, are also good candidates. Women who are planning future pregnancies may be advised to wait, as the vertical muscles in the abdomen that are tightened during surgery will tend to separate again during pregnancy. Men are also candidates for abdominoplasty following massive weight loss or due to aging and lack of exercise. If the fat deposits are all located below the navel, a less complex procedure called a mini-tummy tuck or partial abdominoplasty may be recommended. Both a partial and complete abdominoplasty may be performed in conjunction with liposuction to remove fat deposits from the hips, waist or thighs for a better contour.

Surgical Methods

A tummy tuck is nearly always performed under general anesthesia, but can be performed under local anesthesia with intravenous sedation, epidural anesthesia with sedation, or general anesthesia depending on your health and the extent of the procedure. Some surgeons will perform selected abdominoplasties in an outpatient surgicenter, but most prefer a hospital setting where you can recover overnight.

Full Abdominoplasty: There are several techniques for an abdominoplasty, the most common of which involves an incision made across the lower abdomen, just above the pubic area. This incision can be angled to be easier to conceal. A second incision is usually made to free the navel from surrounding tissue. The surgeon separates the skin from the abdominal wall all the way up to your ribs and lifts a large skin flap to reveal the vertical muscles in your abdomen. These muscles are tightened by pulling them close together and stitching them into their new position. The skin flap is then stretched down and the extra skin is removed. A new opening is made for the belly button at the right position. The incisions are closed with sutures and/or staples, and gauze is placed over the incision area.

Mini Abdominoplasty: In partial or modified tummy tuck, the incision is much shorter and the navel may not need to be moved. The skin is separated only between the incision line and the navel. This skin flap is stretched down, the excess is removed, and the flap is stitched back into place.

Operating Time: 2-5 hours

The Recovery Period

After surgery, you will have soreness and discomfort that can be controlled with medication. You may need to remain in the hospital for two to three days, or hire nursing care at home. When you leave the hospital, the dressing will be replaced with an abdominal supporter that you will be instructed to wear for several weeks. Bed rest is recommended with legs bent at the hips in order to reduce the strain on the abdominal area. You may be up and around in a few days, but avoid straining for three or four weeks. Most people are able to return to work after two to three weeks. You will be given instructions for showering and changing your dressings. At first you may not be able to stand up straight without feeling a tugging sensation, but you should start walking as soon as possible as your body accommodates to your newly tightened abdomen. Postoperative bruising is minimal, but swelling may take up to three months to settle. You may also experience a loss sensation of the abdominal skin that may take several

> *An alternative to tummy tuck could potentially be liposuction. The upper and lower tummy, waist, hips, flanks can be suctioned to reduce girth.*

months to return. Surface stitches will be removed in five to seven days, and deeper sutures, with ends that protrude through the skin, will come out in two to three weeks. Lighter bandages will be applied that will be replaced with an abdominal support garment that is worn for several weeks. If you start out in top physical condition with strong abdominal muscles, recovery from abdominoplasty will be much faster. Moderate exercise will help you heal better, reduce the chance of blood clots and tone muscles. Vigorous exercise should be avoided until you can do it comfortably, at about four to six weeks. It will take nine months to a year before your scars flatten, soften and fade out.

Back to Work: 2-3 weeks

Potential Risks or Side Effects

Possible complications include poor healing, skin loss, asymmetries and the need for a secondary procedure. This surgery does produce a permanent scar, which can extend from hip to hip. The scar can be placed so that it will not show under most clothing including bathing suits. Everyone heals differently and, in some cases, the scar may be thick, raised and irregular. Occasionally, a projection of bulging tissue called a "dog ear" can result which can be easily revised at a later date if necessary. Infections can be treated with drainage and antibiotics, but will prolong your healing process. The risk of blood clots can be minimized by moving around as soon as possible after surgery.

Alternative Treatment Options

An alternative to tummy tuck could potentially be liposuction. The upper and lower tummy, waist, hips, flanks can be suctioned to reduce girth. It is not a substitute for a full tummy tuck, but most patients will get some skin shrinkage. In some cases liposuction will not correct and, in fact, may worsen the appearance of loose skin around the abdomen.

Exercise can dramatically change the appearance of the midriff. The abdominal muscles are considered by most trainers to be one of the easier muscle groups to tone.

Surgical Fee: $4,500-$8,000 plus hospital stay and anesthesia.

chapter 23

*"Looking good has become an informal championship in which
everyone desires to win. Physical beauty is synonymous with
success and likewise unattractiveness spells defeat."*

Welcome to Your Facelift (Doubleday, 1997),
by Helen Bransford

BODY LIFT

Body lifts are ideal for patients who have a significant weight loss and
have been left with unsightly loose pouches of excess skin. It is the most
invasive, yet the most effective technique to restore firm, youthful contours to the body. If you look in the mirror naked, and pull up the saggy
skin of your hips to stretch out your upper thighs and abdominal area,
you can transform the way your body looks. Body lifts are essentially considered "face-lifts for the body." Lower body lifts can address the thighs,
buttocks, abdomen, waist and hips all in one stage. The added benefits
are an overall improvement in dimpling and cellulite, as well as a general pulling up a woman's private parts to a more youthful status. Body lifts
may also be performed after previous liposuction. If there is skin excess
after fat removal, a thigh or body lift may be performed to reduce the
amount of loose tissue. The trade-off is that the recovery is longer than
most other cosmetic surgical procedures and the length of the scarring is
very significant.

Surgical Methods

Body lift surgery is usually performed under general anesthesia because it
is considered major surgery and can be quite extensive. For thigh lifts,
excess skin is lifted and removed through incisions made in the inner thigh
and/or high upper outer thigh. Simultaneous lifting of the thighs and buttocks is done using incisions that follow a high-cut bathing suit line only
a bit higher up on the hip. The surgeon lifts and removes the excess skin
down to the muscle and removes the thick layer of fat beneath the skin.
Drain tubes may be placed at the incision to draw out fluids. The surgery
is often combined with liposuction. The scars can usually be hidden in the

natural skin creases so they are less visible. In some cases a buttock lift may be performed which requires placing scars across the buttock or in the buttock crease.

Operating Time: 3-5 hours

The Recovery Period

The recovery from a body lift procedure is very similar to a tummy tuck. Most patients will stay in the hospital for one to two or more nights after surgery. Keep your head elevated, above the level of your heart, when lying down. Although you may not feel up to it, you should try to walk as soon as possible to reduce swelling and prevent blood clots from forming in your legs. The swelling is mild to moderate and peaks at two to three days. Surgical drains may be placed for several days following the procedure that will have to be emptied. For the first week following surgery you must avoid bending or lifting. Usually the sutures are covered with adhesive steri-strips, tape and surgical gauze. Small amounts of oozing and bleeding are common. Because of the location of the incisions for a thigh lift, it is impossible to avoid lying on them. Changing position at least every 30 minutes and moving around carefully will limit stress on the incision lines. You probably will have several layers of stitches with body lift procedures. Some will be resorbed by the body and some may need to be removed by your surgeon. Deep sutures will be permanent. You usually will be able to shower on the third day after surgery. Moderate pain can be anticipated after this procedure. Numbness in small areas on the thighs is possible but usually disappears gradually over several months. Although most bruising and swelling will disappear within three weeks, some swelling may remain for six months and up to a year. After thigh and buttocks lifts you cannot resume rigorous exercise like jogging or contact sports for approximately six weeks.

Back to Work: 2-3 weeks

Potential Risks or Side Effects

Most lifts require fairly lengthy incisions and scarring is an important consideration. The incisions can usually be hidden under clothing, even some bathing suits. In some patients fluid can collect beneath the skin that may need to be aspirated with a needle. Infection and wound healing complications including skin loss may occur during the first two weeks. Swelling is significant and will take several months to settle fully.

Alternative Treatment Options

A thigh or buttock lift can improve the skin quality and appearance, but cannot eliminate excess fat to the same extent and they are limited in terms of the area treated. A tummy tuck can both remove fat and tighten the skin around the abdomen. Exercise, especially weight lifting, can significantly improve the shape and tone of the body. Liposuction can produce a reduction in size, but liposuction cannot alter skin quality and there may be extra skin once the fat has been removed.

Surgical Fee: $10,000-$15,000 plus hospital stay and anesthesia.

Botox Treatment

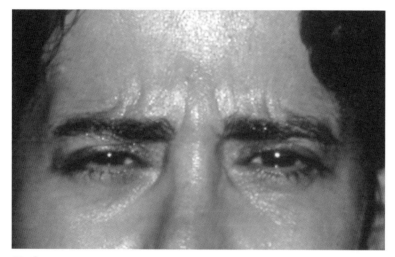

Before

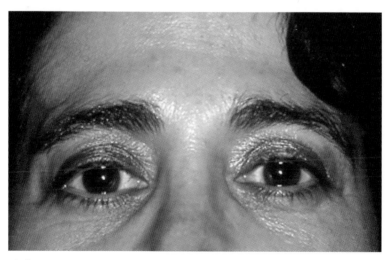

After

Photos courtesy of Marsha Gordon, MD

Breast Surgery: Augmentation

Breast Augmentation

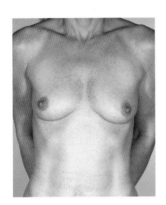
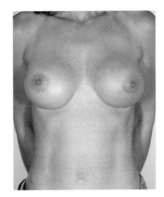

Before   *After*

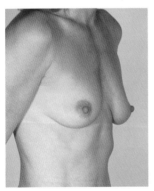
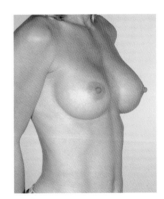

Before   *After*

Photos courtesy of INAMED Aesthetics, Santa Barbara, CA

Breast Reduction

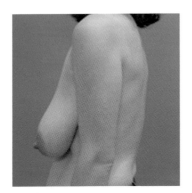

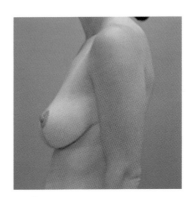

Before   *After*

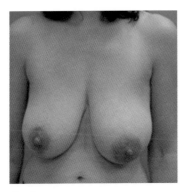

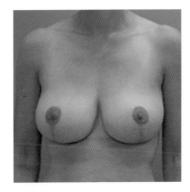

Before   *After*

Photos courtesy of Garth Fisher, MD

Cosmetic Dentistry

Minor orthodontics and tooth whitening

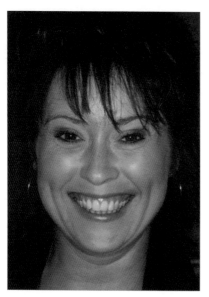 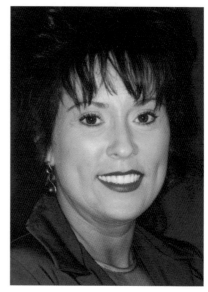

Before　　　　　　　　　　　　　　*After*

She did not like the crowded, crooked and yellowed teeth.

Minor orthodontics with "removable braces" and tooth whitening transformed this smile in only two months

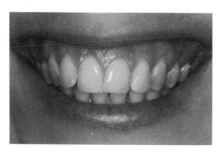 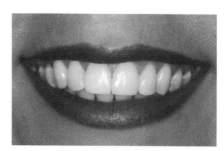

Before　　　　　　　　　　　　　　*After*

Photos courtesy of Michael Malone, DDS

Invisible retainer and porcelain veneers

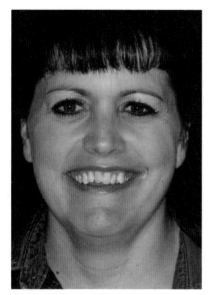 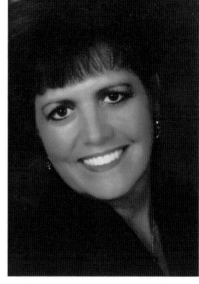

Before   *After*

Poor alignment, dark fillings, and discolored teeth create smile problems for this woman

An invisible retainer to straighten the teeth and porcelain veneers to perfect the smile created a dramatic change.

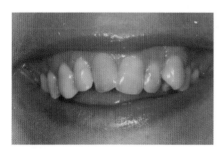 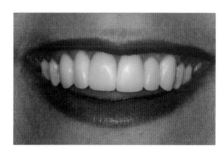

Before   *After*

Photos courtesy of Michael Malone, DDS

Deep Chemical Peels

Phenol Peel

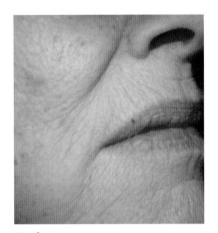
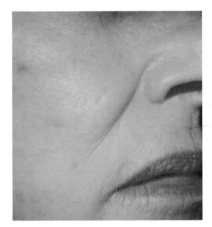

Before   *After*

TCA Peel

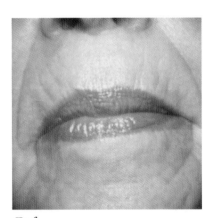
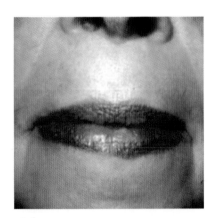

Before   *After*

Photos courtesy of Bruce Katz, MD

Dermal Fillers: Human Collagen

CosmoDerm injection of the lips

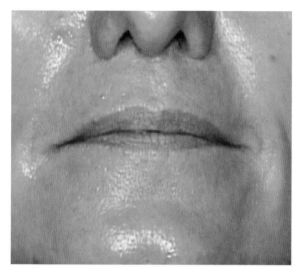

Before

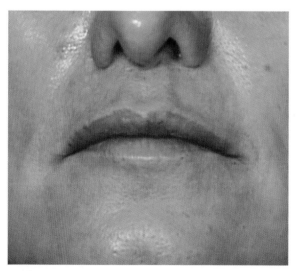

After

Photos courtesy of Tina Alster, MD

Ear Surgery

Otoplasty

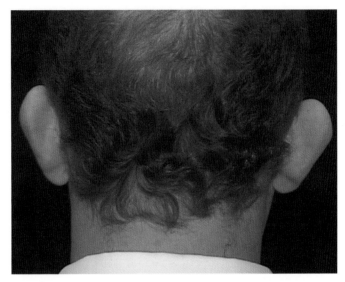

Before

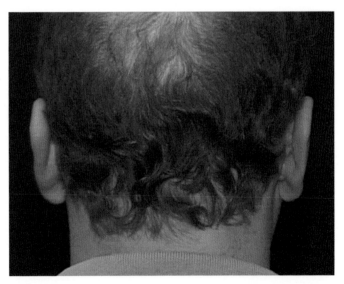

After

Photos courtesy of Malcolm Paul, MD FACS

Blepharoplasty

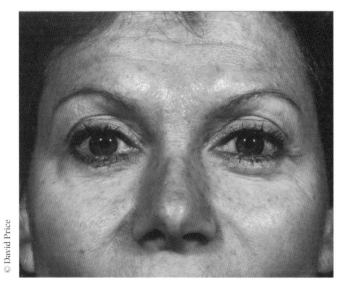

Before

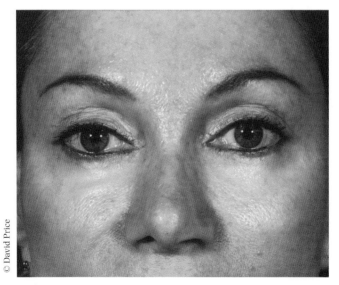

After

Photos courtesy of Z. Paul Lorenc, MD, FACS

Face-lift: Composite

Face-lift, brow lift, chemical peel of lips, and upper eye lid trim

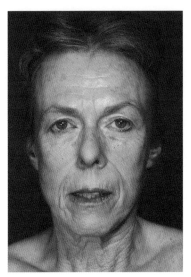

Before

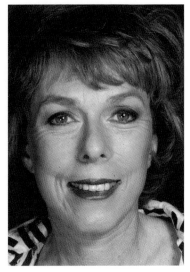

After

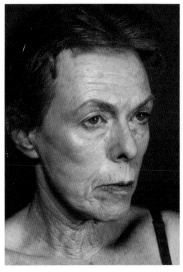

Before

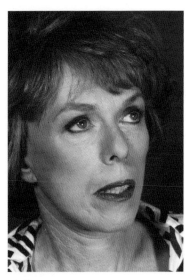

After

Photos courtesy of Gerald H. Pitman, MD, FACS

SMAS face-lift, neck lift, "endoscopic" forehead lift, lower eye lift (blepharoplasty) and fat infections.

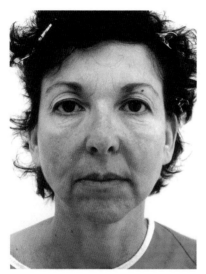

Before

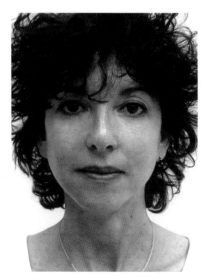

After

Photos courtesy of Timothy J. Marten, MD, FACS

Liposuction

Liposuction of the abdomen

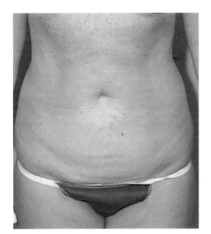

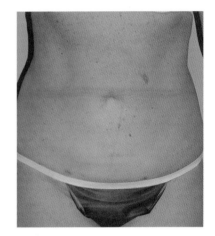

Before

After

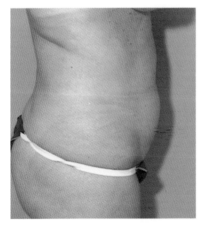

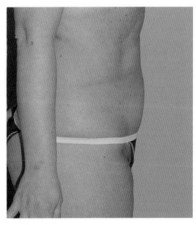

Before

After

Photos courtesy of Robert Bernard, MD, FACS

Liposuction of the hips

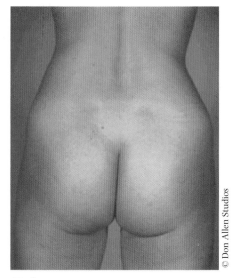

Before

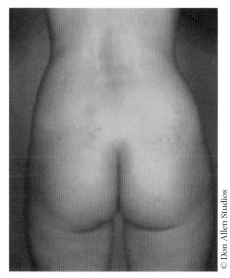

After

Photos courtesy of Alan Matarasso, MD, FACS

Nose Surgery

Rhinoplasty

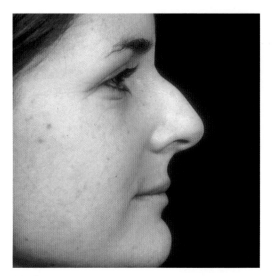

Before

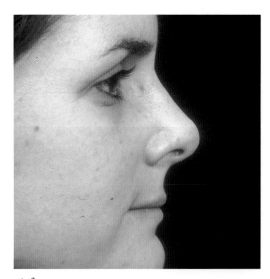

After

Photos courtesy of David Hidalgo, MD

Rhinoplasty

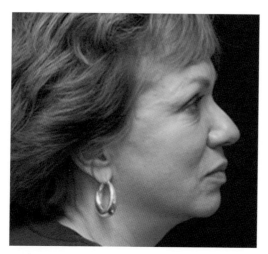

Before

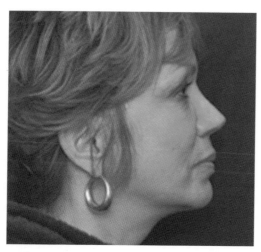

After

Photos courtesy of Alvin Glasgold, MD

Abdominoplasty and Medial Thighplasty

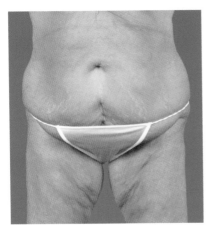 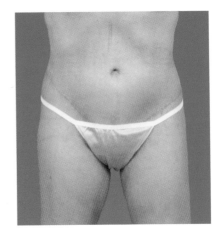

Before   *After*

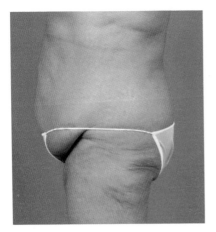 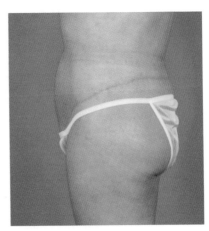

Before   *After*

Photos courtesy of Rod Rohrich, MD, FACS

chapter 24

*"The only parts left of my original body
are my elbows."*

Phyllis Diller

ARM LIFT

The Arm Lift, or Brachioplasty, is performed to surgically eliminate loose, hanging skin from the upper arms. Aging, as well as significant weight loss, can cause skin to become less elastic. Your surgeon will evaluate your upper arms to assess where the fat is located as well as the laxity of our skin. If there is good skin tone, liposuction alone may be recommended. If there is little elasticity left in the skin, an arm lift may be recommended.

Surgical Methods

While you are standing your doctor will mark the area of excess skin to be removed. The incision is usually placed on the inner surface of the upper arm and may extend from the elbow to the armpit; it may be an ellipse or a triangle with the base in the armpit. Incisions are sometimes made on the inner and under surface of the arm in a zigzag pattern. The surgical opening may run from the armpit to as low as the elbow. In some cases, skin excision may be limited to the axillary or underarm area. As the excess skin and fat is removed, the remaining skin is stretched and sutured into place and the incisions are bandaged. Excess skin and fatty tissue are removed. Some fat will be left to cover and protect blood vessels and nerves. The incision is then sutured, and the sutures may or may not be dissolvable. A drain also may be placed to eliminate excess fluid. While you are still in the operating room a compression garment, absorbent bandage, or a simple dressing may be applied. This will help to keep swelling to a minimum.

Operating Time: 1-3 hours

The Recovery Period

During the first week after the procedure keep your upper body propped up and your arms elevated as much as possible. Sleep on a recliner, if possible, or keep pillows behind your back, so you're more sitting than horizontal. If you have to pick something up, bend your knees and squat. Do not lift anything heavier than a phone book. Most doctors advise waiting at least three to four weeks before doing strenuous exercise and six weeks for any upper arm workouts. Some tightness could remain in the area for up to 3 months.

Back to Work: 7-10 days

Potential Risks or Side Effects

The scars from an arm lift are permanently visible. They may appear raised and thickened initially and may take 6-12 months to settle. Women who have had a mastectomy are advised not to have an arm lift. Since the surgery affects the lymphatic drainage, the combined procedures may cause the arm to swell permanently. If you have had phlebitis or inflamed blood vessels in either of your arms, you may not be a candidate for this surgery.

Alternative Treatment Options

Liposuction can be performed to reduce the amount of fatty tissue in the upper arms, but it will not have the same skin tightening effect. If there is some degree of skin elasticity, you may be able to get some improvement from liposuction alone, even though it is not ideal. In some cases liposuction can also be performed on the forearm to reduce the circumference.

Surgical Fee: $2,500-$4,000 plus facility fee and anesthesia

"While cosmetic surgery has been associated almost exclusively with women in the past, in the wake of the enormous explosions of cosmetic surgery interventions, men appear to be altering their appearance is increasing numbers as well."

Dubious Equalities & Embodied Differences (Rowman & Littlefield, 2003)

Kathy Davis

CALF IMPLANTS

Calf implants are used to create the impression of greater definition and contour in the lower leg area. The addition of a calf implant will add width rather than length to the calf area. They are used sometimes to reduce the appearance of bow-leggedness and tibial torsion, which is a twisting below the knees, or to correct an asymmetry that was a result of a congenital deformity or polio.

Surgical Methods

An incision is made below the crease behind the knee. In this position any scar that remains after the surgery most likely will be well concealed; however, the scar will be visible to someone who looks for it. The implant is inserted, and the incision is closed with sutures. The procedure is usually performed in an outpatient surgical center under intravenous sedation. If you are having more than one procedure general anesthesia and overnight hospitalization may be required. Incisions are made in the crease behind the knee and the surgeon creates pockets to hold the implants beneath the fascia. In some cases balloon-like tissue expanders may be used temporarily to allow for gradual stretching of the tissue. After several weeks the expanders are replaced with the implant. If the degree of enlargement is not excessive, the permanent implants are placed immediately. In some cases two implants may need to be placed in each leg. Compression stockings are placed on the calves after the procedure and these will be worn for about two to three weeks.

Operating Time: 1-3 hours

The Recovery Period

Bed rest immediately following surgery is recommended as calves will feel stiff and sore. After 24 hours you can get up to eat or go to the bathroom, although you will have to avoid climbing stairs. Keeping the legs elevated will reduce the swelling and therefore reduce pain. You can expect to feel as if you have had an intense calf workout that lasts for two weeks. You will need to be off your feet for about a week and sleep on your back for at least 10 days to allow for proper healing without pocket disruption. Only low heeled shoes should be worn right after surgery. Your sutures on the exterior may be of the dissolving or non-dissolving type. Non-dissolving sutures will be removed in approximately 10 days. You must be careful not to strain the muscles in that area or lift heavy objects that affect your calf muscles for several weeks to avoid disrupting the implant. As you resume walking, it is normal to feel some discomfort until the swelling resolves. Most people find walking on their toes or in shoes with heels the most comfortable during this healing phase. Avoid strenuous use of the legs for at least six weeks to allow for healing and to make sure the implant has securely positioned itself. Upper body workouts can be resumed in a week; light leg workouts can begin in three weeks.

Sometimes calf implants can shift slightly out of alignment and a second operation may be necessary to reposition the implants.

Back to Work: 10-14 days

Potential Risks or Side Effects

Possible complications include extrusion of the implant works its way back up to the skin's surface, capsular contracture, which is an excess tightening of the scar tissue that may distort the implant, and asymmetry. If an infection occurs the implant might have to be temporarily removed and replaced at a later time. In rare instances the blood supply may become compromised, and can result in gangrene, which is a serious complication. Sometimes calf implants can shift slightly out of alignment and a second operation may be necessary to reposition the implants. Temporary loss of sensitivity is to be expected. There will be a permanent scar behind the knee. During the recovery there is also a risk of the implant becoming distorted as the body heals around it. In very rare cases the implant may weaken the nearby muscle.

Alternative Treatment Options

Although there are no other procedures that will enlarge the calf, exercise, especially weight lifting and cycling, should always be considered an alternative to surgery for building up the calves.

Surgical Fee: The price for calf implants is approximately $5,000 plus hospital stay and anesthesia.

section IV

PARA-SURGICAL PROCEDURES

There are a wide array of non-surgical treatments available that can be performed to improve your appearance, soften lines and wrinkles, plump up facial contours, and minimize skin conditions like acne, rosacea and hyperpigmentation. These treatments can be considered alternatives to going under the knife, or as adjuncts to cosmetic surgery that enhance and maintain the results. Scientific advancements are responsible for the introduction of new technologically-driven methods that are increasingly less invasive and produce visible results without some of the down-time, discomfort and costs of more invasive treatments. The advent of botulinum toxin for cosmetic uses and laser therapies for the skin is widely considered to have revolutionized the field of cosmetic medicine over the past decade. This section will cover some of the most popular of the para-surgical procedures and discuss some of the developments we can expect to hear more about in the next few years.

chapter 26

"If a woman's face is her fortune — it now costs a fortune. $20,000 and up, depending on how much gets lifted."

Dodie Goes Shopping (St Martin's Press, 1999)
by Dodie Kazanjian

DERMAL FILLERS

Soft tissue fillers involve injecting or implanting a substance under the skin to plump up, or contour, and soften wrinkles, furrows, scars and hollows in the face. Filling substances may include bovine collagen, hyaluronic acid gel, liquid silicone, fat removed from another part of your body, and many other variations, as well as polymer implants. The wide array of choices in filling materials makes this area of cosmetic medicine very controversial. All doctors have their favorite techniques, and most doctors offer several different types of fillers in their practice. Not every filling substance is right for every face or function, and doctors like to use a wide spectrum of choices that are suitable for different purposes. Generally, thicker substances are best for deeper creases and recontouring areas like cheek hollows and lips. Thinner substances work better for fine lines and superficial wrinkles or in areas where the skin is thin like around the eyelids and the lip lines. Each filler is injected in a unique manner, and there is a learning curve to getting the technique just right. Treatments may often vary from one doctor to another.

Read the product literature in advance or check out the company's website for details about any filler you are considering. It is also a good idea to keep your own records of what type of treatment you had, when you had it, and how much was used. Most doctors will record this in your medical chart so that they know how much they injected into each area. In this way, when you return for a touch up, the doctor can judge how well the material lasted and decide to use more if needed for maximum correction. It may be recommended that you return in two to three weeks after treatment for a touch-up in case any refinements are needed.

In some cases laser skin resurfacing, microdermabrasion or peels may be more effective than adding volume to the face, because they soften wrinkles by removing and smoothing the outer layers of the skin. There is a common misconception that botulinum toxin is a wrinkle filler. Rather, it is a muscle blockade that is injected in very tiny amounts into specific muscles to treat and improve lines, wrinkles and furrows associated with facial expression. Since the advent of botulinum toxin in facial rejuvenation, dermal fillers are used less frequently for the forehead and around the eyes. If the creases between the brows are very deep, a filler could be used to smooth it, but botulinum toxin is usually the first course of treatment. The botulinum toxin in this instance is preventative, and the filler substance is a corrective measure.

Questions to ask your doctor before having a dermal filler treatment

- What is the source of the material?
- Is it natural or synthetic?
- How long has it been on the market?
- How long has the doctor been using it?
- What is the name of the manufacturer and where are they located?
- What kinds of clinical studies have been done?
- What are the possible side effects?
- Do I need a skin test before treatment?
- Could I be allergic to it?
- What does a reaction look like and how long does it last?
- What can be done if I have a reaction to it?
- How many treatments will I need and how often?
- How much will each treatment cost?
- If it doesn't look right, what can be done to remove it?
- Can I still have other fillers later on?
- Is it FDA-approved?
- If not, is the company planning to apply for FDA approval in the near future?
- Is it an off-label use?

Dermal Fillers Can be
Classified in Two Ways

Resorbable Fillers: Made from natural or synthetic materials that are broken down and resorbed by the body over time. They are temporary and will need to be repeated, typically in three to nine months on average. The good news is that if you are not happy with the results, it will eventually disappear. If you have treatments with resorbable fillers, you can usually have another filler injected in the same area at a later date. Of these, hyaluronic acid is quickly gaining recognition as one of the most promising.

Nonresorbable Fillers: These contain synthetic components that are not broken down by the body. They are considered permanent because the particles cannot be removed, or 'semi permanent' because the particles are suspended in a substance that gets absorbed in three to six months. They are considered permanent because some of the material cannot be removed after it has been injected. The term "permanent" can be somewhat misleading. As the aging process continues, you will need additional treatments.

Potential Risks or Side Effects

New dermal fillers continue to be under clinical investigation all the time, and products with a high incidence of reactions and complications tend to have difficulty getting approved by the FDA. However, Europe, South America and other parts of the world have less stringent criteria and fillers are often approved for medical and cosmetic use based on unsubstantiated clinical data. The duration of dermal fillers is variable and depends on the formulation of the material, how deeply it is injected, how much is used as well as how severe the wrinkles or folds are. Most dermal fillers are only temporarily effective so that repeat treatments will be needed every three to six months on average. There may be bruising and swelling following any dermal filler treatment. Itching and mild discomfort are not uncommon. Asymmetries, hardening and lumps are also potential complications. Some substances, such as bovine collagen, require pre-treatment testing for allergic reactions. Although less than three percent of people are allergic to bovine collagen, a reaction may cause itching, hives, redness and prolonged swelling. With a few exceptions, most commercially available filling substances have no anesthetic added, making them somewhat painful to have injected. Topical anesthetic agents are often used for numbing and a dental or lip block may be needed for very sensitive areas like the lips and around the mouth.

Post Procedure

Recovery time will depend on the extent of the treatment and how much material is injected. Most people experience some swelling and redness for the first 24-48 hours. When large amounts of any substance are injected into the face, swelling may last from several days to one week. Most injectable fillers have short recovery periods and you can return to work the same day or the next day. Some people swell more than others and bruising is common, but can be covered with camouflage makeup as needed. In more extensive procedures, such as fat injections into multiple areas, local anesthesia or light sedation may be required.

The following list is by no means complete. We have identified the most common products used in the U.S. at the time of printing. At last count, there are more than 70 commercially available fillers reportedly on the market around the world, most of which will never enter into widespread use and will not enter the FDA approval process for various reasons including safety record and lack of funding.

A Word About Food and Drug Administration Approval

Many products and drugs are used in the cosmetic field even though they may not have FDA approval for a specific cosmetic indication. This does not necessarily constitute an illegal use of an approved substance. A physician may obtain access to an unapproved drug by participating in a clinical study as an investigator.

In some cases, "off label" use means that the drug or filler is approved for a use other than facial wrinkles. For example, botulinum toxin type A only recently got FDA approval for the application of facial glabellar wrinkles, although it has been widely used for cosmetic purposes for more than a decade in the U.S.

COMMON DERMAL FILLERS

ANIMAL-DERIVED

Bovine collagen	Zyplast ®, Zyderm®
Hyaluronic acid gel	Hylaform®, Hylaform Plus®, Hylaform Fine®

NON-ANIMAL

Hyaluronic acid gel	Restylane®, Restylane Fine®, Perlane®

HUMAN TISSUES

Derived from human cadaveric tissues from a tissue bank or autologous tissues taken from your own body.

AUTOLOGOUS

Fat

TISSUE BANKS:

Fascialata	Fascian®
Dermis	Cymetra®, AlloDerm®

HUMAN COLLAGEN:

Fibroblasts	CosmoDerm™, CosmoPlast™

SEMI-PERMANENT

Bovine collagen with PMMA	ArteColl® or ArteFill®
Hydroxyl Apatite	Radiance™

PERMANENT

Liquid silicone	Silikon 1000, SilSkin®

RESORBABLE FILLING SUBSTANCES

Autologous Fat

Fat is perhaps the most widespread material used as a filling substance in facial rejuvenation. The fat that is injected into facial areas comes from your own body so there is no chance of an allergic reaction. Fat can be used in higher volumes than most other injectable materials and can be used to create a fuller, more youthful appearance by reestablishing pleasing contours. Injections of fat into the deep layers of facial tissue can soften the angular, thin appearance that often accompanies aging. Fat is the first choice of material when injections of larger volumes greater than 10cc are needed. The procedure is a two-step process that usually requires several treatments. The fat must be harvested from your own body, typically from the abdomen, thighs or hips. After it is extracted it is placed in a centrifuge to separate the fat from surrounding tissues. The fat is then packed into a syringe ready to be injected. Because fat molecules are somewhat larger than other injectable materials, it is usually injected more deeply and with a larger gauge needle. Larger volumes of up to 50 -100 cc's, or roughly a third-of-a-cup, can be used over the entire face at one stage. It can be particularly useful around the mouth, hollows around eyelids, cheeks, depressions, scars, lips, and in the hands.

Duration: Fat injections have a variable life span. Much of the fat may be absorbed within six months. The fat is slowly absorbed by the body, although the amount of absorption varies by individual and is hard to predict. Typically, more than half of the fat used in injectable treatments is absorbed within six months of the operation, although it may last longer. Almost all patients will permanently retain some of the injected fat. Follow-up treatments are usually advised.

Bovine Collagen

More than one million treatments worldwide have been performed and bovine collagen remains the most widely used dermal filler on the market. Zyderm® and Zyplast® (Inamed Corp) are composed of highly purified bovine dermal collagen that has been used to correct facial imperfections since the 1980s. The bovine collagen is processed to create a product that is similar to human collagen. There are three forms: Zyderm 1®, Zyderm 2®, and Zyplast®. Four weeks prior to the procedure a test dose is administered in the forearm to determine if a patient has a sensitivity to the implant material. Three percent of people tested may have sensitivities. Frequently, a second test dose is administered. Collagen is most commonly used to fill out superficial wrinkles, skin depressions and some scars.

> *One of the fascinating categories of filling agents is derived from human tissue. Most of these products are obtained from cadaver tissue through tissue banks.*

Duration: 2-6 months

Hyaluronic Acid Gel

Hyaluronic acid is a natural polysaccharide that is commonly found in the connective tissues of the body. The source of the material can be from animals (avian protein; i.e., roosters or poultry), or bacterial fermentation which is non-animal. Its normal function in the body is to bind water and to lubricate moving parts like joints. The most common areas for treatment are the naso-labial folds (creases from the nose to mouth), the naso-mental creases (corners of the mouth) and around the lips, as well as cheek and chin contours. Since there is no anesthetic supplied in the syringe, some pain relief is needed to keep the patient comfortable, especially in the lip area which is more tender. Aside from expected temporary redness/puffiness for the first day or two, there are few complications to report. The longevity of a treatment can be four to six months and even longer in some patients. Hyaluronic acid gel formulas come preloaded in syringes, without the benefit of Lidocaine or local anesthetic. As the substance naturally occurs in humans, allergic reactions are rare. Many varieties of hyaluronic acid gel are being used in Canada and Europe. At the time of printing, none of these fillers is approved by the FDA for cosmetic use in the U.S. Restylane® (Q-Med/Medicis) is pending approval and it is widely expected that this product will be available in the U.S. by the end of 2003.

Duration: 4-12 months

Polylactic Acid

Developed by a French dermatologist, New-Fill® is based on a substance called "polylactic acid" (PLA) which occurs naturally and has been used in suture material for years. PLA stimulates production of the body's own collagen within the line or wrinkle, making the skin appear smoother and firmer. New-Fill® has to be reconstituted to be injected and is most commonly used in the lips, nasal labial folds, cheek hollows and scars. The substance is non-allergenic and typically two to three treatment sessions are recommended for best results. At the time of printing, New-Fill® is entering clinical trials in the U.S. for approval, and is available in Europe and elsewhere around the world.

Duration: 6-12 months

Human Tissues

One of the fascinating categories of filling agents is derived from human tissue. Most of these products are obtained from cadaver tissue through tissue banks. Donor suitability is determined according to the standards of the American Association of Tissue Banks (MTB) and FDA. Cadaver collagen must meet criteria established for extensive testing for human immunodeficiency virus antibody (HIV), Hepatitis B, Hepatitis C and syphilis.

Cosmoderm™/Cosmoplast™

A new human tissue filler that received approval in March 2003 is marketed under the name of CosmoDerm™ and CosmoPlast™ (Inamed Corp). It contains human collagen that has been purified from a single fibroblast cell culture. This product does contain 0.3% Lidocaine, so additional local anesthesia is usually not required. No skin test is needed because it is fashioned from human tissues rather than an animal source. CosmoDerm™ and CosmoPlast™ are injected just below the surface of the skin to fill in superficial lines and wrinkles and to define the border of the lips.

Duration: 2-6 months

Fascian™

Fascian™ is an injectable form of preserved fascia. Fascia are sheets of thick connective tissue layers that wrap around most of the internal structures of the body, including the muscles. Fascian™ is produced from fascia lata, the thick sheet of fascia from along the outer side of the thigh muscle, and supplied in an injectable form. Once it is injected into an area, the liquid in the suspension is absorbed and the residual particles fill the defect. Fascian™ comes in a freeze-dried form in a variety of particle sizes that can be used to treat problems of different size and type, such as acne scars. It is rehydrated by adding Lidocaine or a similar injection solution into the syringe. Fascian™ may feel thick or lumpy in the area, especially during the initial period after injection. Although bruising is possible, infection and local reaction are rare. Some degree of reabsorption of the material is to be expected.

Duration: up to 2 years

AlloDerm®/Cymetra™

AlloDerm® is human dermal tissue that has been decellularized to remove the risk of rejection or inflammation. It comes in strips in a freeze dried form to be implanted into lips, nasal defects and around the eyelids. AlloDerm® is sometimes used as a soft-tissue replacement in facial reconstruction to build up cheeks, chins, hollows and asymmetries. It can be rolled or layered so that it can be implanted under the skin to fill out depressions. Cymetra™ was introduced in 2000. It is Micronized AlloDerm® Tissue in an injectable form. It also needs to be reconstituted. More than one treatment may be required to achieve the level of correction envisioned.

Duration: AlloDerm® may last up to 2 years; Cymetra™ may last 2-4 months

NON-RESORBABLE FILLING SUBSTANCES

Artecoll® (Artefill®)

ArteColl® is a semi-permanent filler currently used in Europe, Canada and Mexico. It is made up of 75% percent bovine collagen and 25% polymethyl-methacrylate microspheres (PMMA) which are carbon-based polymers. PMMA has been used in dental work, hip prostheses and bone cement. The product is mixed with a local anesthetic, Lidocaine, to numb the area to be injected. Over three months the collagen fibers get absorbed, leaving the PMMA behind, which is too large to be broken down and remains permanently. It is tunneled under the skin, massaged and molded to fill the area to be treated. ArteColl® can be used for acne scars, nasolabial folds, and for filling depressions such as sunken cheeks. Possible complications include lumping, inflammation, granulomas or localized hardening, rash, and the migration of the microspheres into other areas. Because of its permanence, ArteColl® requires greater skill to inject and may be more risky than other biological fillers.

> *Not all forms of silicone are created equal. It varies by degree of purity, and "non-injectable" grade silicone has been very problematic when used to treat facial lines.*

Duration: Collagen resorbs in 3 months, PMMA particles are permanent

Radiance™

Radiance™ (BioForm) is composed of calcium hydroxyl apatite, which has been used in the body for multiple applications including cheek and chin implants. Radiance™ is injected into the face adding volume through microspheres that are suspended in polysaccharide carriers until encapsulation occurs. CA Hydroxyl apatite has been used for many years for other medical purposes in both injectable and solid implant forms, such as facial reconstruction. Radiance™ is FDA approved only for vocal cord paralysis and urinary incontinence. However, off-label use is permitted in the U.S. Radiance™ is a pure, synthetic calcium hydroxyl apatite composed of calcium and phosphate ions which occur naturally in the body so they are biocompatible. The particles are in a gel carrier made up of cellulose, glycerin and purified water. The product manufacturer claims that Radiance™ will remain soft and pliable as it permeates soft, fibrous tissue. As with any long term filling agent, there is a possibility of a foreign body reaction which can cause lumps or granulomas, and migration.

Duration: 2+ years

Injectable Silicone

Not all forms of silicone are created equal. It varies by degree of purity, and "non-injectable" grade silicone has been very problematic when used to treat facial lines. The form that is making a comeback in the US is sterile, purified, medical injectable grade silicone. The newest method of injection is referred to as the "micro droplet" technique, which has the advantage of causing fewer hard lumps than previous variations. Liquid silicone is only approved by the FDA for ophthalmic uses, so applying it for cosmetic purposes is considered an off label use of an approved product. There are instances where injectable silicone may be very beneficial, such as acne scars, nasal and chin defects, or for older patients where the long term effects are less of a concern.

Duration: Permanent

Fees: Fees for dermal fillers vary based on the number of the areas that are treated and the type and amount of material used. Autologous fat is perhaps the most variable, because it is a two stage procedure. The costs for fat injections typically range from $500 and up to $5,000, depending on the extent of the areas to be injected and whether fat is stored between treatments. Most dermal filler treatments are priced by the number of syringes used. Commercially available fillers, with few exceptions, come in pre-loaded syringes that range from 0.4cc, to 1.0 or 2.0 cc's. Fees may be based on the number of syringes used; for example, the first cc may cost $500, and the second cc may cost $400. A standard treatment is usually more than just one syringe. You should know before you have your treatment how much the doctor estimates the total cost to be. If you are on a budget, tell the doctor that you are only able to spend a certain amount on your treatment so he can gauge the amount he will inject accordingly. You can always go back for more.

"One brow wrinkle is the result of 200,000 frowns."

"Real Facts" at Snapple.com

BOTULINUM TOXIN

Botulinum toxin was originally used to treat eye spasms and central nervous system disorders. Since the late 1980s it has been used for cosmetic purposes, as well as medical therapies. Botulinum toxin A, a purified protein made from botulism bacteria, binds to the nerve endings preventing the release of the chemical transmitters that activate muscles. When injected into specific areas of the face it paralyzes the small muscles that cause frown lines, crow's feet and other wrinkles. Botulinum Toxin treatment decreases muscle activity thereby preventing the appearance of "dynamic" wrinkles that are caused by repeated facial expressions. The toxin acts on the junctions between nerves and muscles, preventing the release of a chemical messenger called acetylcholine from the nerve endings. Tiny amounts are injected into a specific facial muscle so only the targeted impulse of that muscle will be blocked, causing a local relaxation. It acts as a muscle block to immobilize the underlying cause of the unwanted lines caused by muscle contractions and to prevent wrinkle formation. Since the muscles can no longer make the offending facial expression, the lines gradually smooth out from disuse and new creases are prevented from forming. Other muscles that are not treated are not affected so a natural look and expressions are maintained. Botox may not be as effective on lines that are not entirely caused by the action of a muscle, i.e. the nasal labial folds that are formed by a combination of muscle action and the weight of sagging skin. Treatment of some areas is less effective because the muscles are needed for expression and important functions like eating, kissing and opening the eyes. For deeper wrinkles a combination of Botulinum Toxin and a filler, such as fat or hyaluronic acid gel, is sometimes recommended.

Botulinum Toxin is considered to be most effective when administered around the eyes and forehead, but other areas of the face and neck can be treated. The effect generally lasts from four to six months. Some studies indicate that after multiple treatments results can last longer in between treatments. Every person responds differently and different areas tend to have longer lasting results than other areas of the face and neck. Typically the frowning area lasts the longest, whereas areas around the mouth last the least long.

The procedure is usually performed in your doctor's office and takes between 15-30 minutes. First, the skin may be treated with a topical anesthetic, if requested. A thin, fine-gauge needle is then used to inject the Botulinum Toxin into the skin and muscle of a specific part of the face. Some physicians use a needle connected to an EMG or electromyography recorder to guide them to target the most active part of the muscle. Crow's feet are treated with three or more injections on the side of the face close to the outer eye area or orbital rim. Forehead creases are typically treated with 10 to 16 small injections, thereby weakening rather than paralyzing the forehead muscles. Botulinum Toxin can be used to improve the appearance of naso-labial folds between the nose and lips, and the fine lines above the lips. Vertical muscle bands in the neck can also be effectively treated with Botulinum Toxin.

BOTULINUM TOXIN USES

- Vertical lines between the brows
- Lines at the bridge of the nose
- Crow's-feet or squint lines
- Horizontal forehead lines
- Muscle bands on the neck
- Under eyelid creases
- Uneven eyebrows
- Popply or cobblestone chin
- Chin creases
- Drooping corners of the mouth
- Upper lip lines
- Muscle roll under the eyes
- Décolleté lines
- Migraine headaches
- Palms and soles for excessive sweating

Forms of Botulinum Toxin

There are various strains of botulinum toxin and Type A is considered the most potent and the most commonly used. Currently BOTOX COSMETIC® is the only form of Botulinum Toxin approved by the FDA for cosmetic purposes. Two others forms, Myobloc® and Dysport®, are currently under FDA review.

Type A: (BOTOX COSMETIC®, Dysport®) Botulinum Toxin Type A purified neurotoxin complex has been used since 1980 to treat muscle disorders, such as lazy eye, eye ticks and uncontrolled blinking. This form has to be reconstituted with normal saline before use. BOTOX COSMETIC® received approval for cosmetic use from the FDA in the spring of 2002 for glabellar creases. Approval for Dysport® is still pending with the FDA.

> *Currently BOTOX COSMETIC® is the only form of Botulinum Toxin approved by the FDA for cosmetic purposes.*

Type B: (Myobloc®) Botulinum Toxin Type B has been introduced more recently. It is in use outside U.S. and is FDA approved only for cervical dystonias, a neurological disorder and not cosmetic uses. This form comes as a pre-made liquid that does not require a diluting agent. Compared with Type A, it has a longer shelf life of up to two years, requires a larger dose, works somewhat faster, but is also slightly more painful when injected.

Post Procedure

Although there is some discomfort involved with the injections, the feeling is much like any other injection and there is virtually no pain afterwards. The treatment can sometimes cause a brief headache and bruising can occur at the injection site. Applying ice packs over the treated site before and after the injections can reduce the discomfort, swelling and bruising. You can go back to work and resume regular activities immediately after the treatment. It is important, however, to keep the head upright for four to six hours and to avoid touching or massaging the treated area. Repeated contraction of the muscles treated can speed the absorption of the Botulinum Toxin. Although Botulinum Toxin injections can have a dramatic effect on dynamic wrinkles, while preventing further wrinkling, it has no overall effect on the texture of the skin.

Risks or Potential Side Effects

The number one risk that most people fear is a droopy eyelid, which is rare. This occurs in less than one-half of one percent of the time. Certain risk factors can predispose you to having this reaction, such as having a low brow position. A drooping eyelid or ptosis is temporary but can take up to six weeks to disappear. In some cases, you may be given prescription eye drops to speed-up the process. Typically, the droop appears about five days after injection. It may start with a slight droopiness at the beginning, progressing to being noticeably droopy for a few days, and then gradually gets better until it is gone. The whole cycle may last ten days. Some people complain of a slight headache after injection. The effects of Botulinum Toxin treatment are not permanent and are reversible. Botulinum Toxin is used in higher doses in deeper muscles of the neck, and it is rare but possible to have difficulty swallowing temporarily after having a treatment in the neck. Anyone who has a neuromuscular disorder such as myasthenia gravis, or who has been on amino glycoside antibiotics, may be advised not to have Botulinum toxin injections. Women who are pregnant, nursing, or who are trying to become pregnant, may be advised not to be treated.

Duration: It takes two to ten days to achieve the full effect. In most cases the treatment lasts for 4 to 6 months. There is evidence that in some cases the more treatments you have, the longer the injections will last between treatments.

Fees: Botulinum Toxin injections vary in cost according to the individual physician and where he or she practices. The average cost in the US per injection site is $350. A treatment of the forehead and crow's feet may range from $600 to $1,500 depending on the amount used and the geographic region you are in.

chapter 28

"Skin rejuventation procedure volume is forecast to grow to more than 29 million annual treatments in 2007, generating approximately $2.9 billion in fees. Wrinkle removal treatment volume is expected to reach 5.6 million procedures producing $4.2 billion in fees by 2007."

Medical Insight Inc., July 2003
Michael Moretti

RESURFACING

The term resurfacing is used to describe a wide range of skin treatments, from chemical to manual physical exfoliation. The procedure improves skin imperfections by peeling away the skin's outer layers. Chemical peels

Questions To Ask Before Having a Skin Resurfacing Procedure

- Is this the most effective treatment for my skin type and condition?
- Is my skin type appropriate for this type of treatment?
- What are the possible side effects?
- How long lasting are the results?
- How many treatments will I need?
- How often should I have a treatment?
- What will happen if I stop having treatments?
- What is the recovery process?
- When can I wear makeup?
- When can I start using my normal skin care regimen again?
- Is there anything I should be using on my skin before the treatment?
- Are intravenous sedation or local anesthesia necessary?
- Is this treatment best done during the winter or when I will not be outdoors?
- Who will be administering my treatment and what are his/her qualifications?

vary according to their active ingredients, their strength, how long the solution remains on the skin, and the pH. Diverse types of peeling agents penetrate to different levels and, consequently produce varying results. They are all similar in that they involve applying a chemical solution to remove damaged outer layers of skin so that newer layers can replace the old ones. A chemical peel can resurface skin to reduce wrinkles and fine lines around the eyes and mouth, sun spots, age spots, freckles, blotchy skin, mild scarring, some types of acne, and actinic keratoses or precancerous lesions. Chemical peels can be an excellent maintenance treatment following more extensive procedures like a face-lift, brow lift or eyelid surgery, or laser resurfacing.

"Personal beauty is a greater recommendation than any letter of reference."

Aristotle, BC 384-322, Greek Philosopher

PEELS

Your doctor will give you specific instructions to prepare for a resurfacing procedure. You may be prescribed medications to take prior to the treatment to prevent a bacterial infection and topical medications to prepare the skin and decrease the risk of pigmentation changes. You must be free of active skin infections, including acne and any type of cold sore, including herpes simplex. You must also not have taken Accutane® for a period of 12-18 months before a treatment, depending on your doctor's specifications. You will be asked to limit your sun exposure at least a month before the peel. You should wear loose clothing that to put on over your head, and refrain from wearing makeup or shaving on the day of treatment, and waxing facial areas for several days or weeks. Darker skin poses special considerations due to increased risk of undesirable skin pigmentation changes.

The surgeon selects the best chemical or chemical mix for you. A solution is applied using a sponge, cotton pad, swab or brush to the areas to be treated. The deeper a peel penetrates, the more visible results you can achieve, but the lengthier the recovery period may be. Most peels can be performed on the face, neck, chest, hands, arms and legs. Your doctor may use a combination of chemicals for your procedure to tailor the treatment specifically to your skin type and condition. A peel treatment begins with cleansing the skin and removing all traces of grease with rubbing alcohol or acetone. The face is then rinsed with water and dried with a small fan. The doctor applies the peeling agent so that all areas of the skin to be treated are covered evenly. A grey-white film, referred to as "frost", develops on the skin by the end of the application. The peeling solution is left in place for a few minutes and then thoroughly neutralized or removed with water.

TYPES OF CHEMICAL PEELS

TYPE	RESULTS	PEEL SOLUTIONS	ANESTHESIA
Superficial Peels	Short-term	AHA, BHA	No
Medium Peels	Intermediate	Jessner's Solution, TCA	Not usually
Deep Peels	Long-term	Phenol, TCA Peels	Intravenous sedation

Types of Chemical Peels

Superficial Peels: The most commonly preformed chemical peels are superficial. These peels use mild chemical solutions like glycolic acid, lactic acid, and salicylic acid to lightly peel the skin with almost no recovery involved. They are typically done in a series to maintain results over time and light peels performed in the physician's office require no anesthesia and the process usually takes 10 to 20 minutes. Your face may be seem slightly red and you can expect the redness to be followed by temporary flaking, dryness and scaling until your skin adjusts to the treatments. Superficial peels are usually combined with an at home skin care regimen for best results. The solution used will typically be adjusted for each treatment session based on your skin's response.

Medium Peels: Jessner's Solution, Trichloroacetic Acid (TCA) or other solutions are used to correct pigment problems, superficial blemishes, moderate sun damage, fine lines and weathered skin. TCA peels are performed in a doctor's office. Anesthesia is usually not necessary because the chemical solution actually numbs the skin. You may feel a warm or burning sensation which is followed by some stinging. Your doctor will control the depth to which the chemical penetrates. In some cases, pre treatment with Retin-A® or bleaching agents like Hydroquinone may be recommended to prevent skin discoloration post peel.

Deep Peels: Phenol and croton oil peels are usually one-time procedure. They can produce more dramatic, long-term results on wrinkles, brown age spots, mild scarring and pre-cancerous growths. Because phenol peels result in permanently lighter skin, they are not recommended for darker skin tones and require that sunscreen be used at all times afterwards. Phenol peels are usually performed in a doctor's office or surgi-center. A full-face, deep chemical peel requires intravenous sedation. You will be monitored with an EKG during a deep chemical peel. You may feel a warm or burning sensation which is followed by some stinging. A full-face phenol peel generally takes one or two hours, while a phenol peel to a smaller area on the face, such as the upper lip, may take only 15 minutes.

Micro-Dermabrasion

Micro-dermabrasion is considered a peel alternative. It entails blasting the face with sterile micro-particles to rub off the very top skin layer, then vac-uuming out the particles and the dead skin. Through a wand-like hand piece, tiny aluminum oxide or salt crystals are delivered at high velocity onto the skin surface and immediately vacuumed away with the same instrument, taking the top-most layer of dead skin cells with it. The tech-nique exfoliates and gently resurfaces the skin, promoting the formation of new smoother skin. It is usually performed on the face and neck, but can be performed on any part of the body including the hands, chest, arms and legs. Micro-dermabrasion can improve rough skin texture, some types of mild scarring, uneven pigmentation and superficial brown spots. It is also useful for acne lesions, blackheads, some stretch marks and fine wrinkles. One of the main advantages of micro-dermabrasion is that it can be safely used for all skin types. The results are similar to a light chemical peel with minimal discomfort, no need for anesthesia, and little or no downtime. The procedure is simple; goggles are placed over your eyes to protect them and the skin is cleansed. Tiny crystals are sprayed on the skin and suctioned back up into the machine. The pressure can be varied to control the amount of penetration or pass over an area several times to remove the most dam-aged skin. Each treatment will take 20-30 minutes. A typical regimen con-sists of a series of four to eight treatments done at intervals of two to four weeks. Immediately after the procedure, makeup can be applied. The skin will have a pink glow that will fade within a few hours. Micro-dermabra-sion can improve the texture of the skin and can be combined with other resurfacing procedures such as chemical peels and laser resurfacing.

Post Procedure

Superficial peels and micro-dermabrasion treatments require little or no downtime. After the procedure, the skin may be coated with a mild ointment. For medium and deep peels your doctor may recommend a soft diet and suggest that you rest and minimize talking and chewing for a few days. A mild pain medication may also be prescribed for deeper peels. Swelling and crusting of the skin are to be expected. You may be given an ointment to apply to your skin for seven to 10 days following the peel to keep it supple and to prevent scabbing. A TCA peel usually results in swelling and blisters that scab over. Most people can resume their normal activities in 7-10 days when the new skin has emerged. At the end of a deep peel, the treated skin may be coated with petroleum jelly or a dressing, which will be left on a day or two. If you have had your face peeled your eyes may swell shut and you will need to have someone to care for you for 48 hours after the procedure. With all peels it is important to avoid sun exposure for several months to protect the newly formed layers of skin. Chlorinated pools should be avoided for a month or so. With a phenol peel new skin will begin to form in about seven to ten days. Your face will be very red at first, gradually fading to a pinkish color over the following weeks. After about two weeks your skin will be healed enough that you can resume normal activities and begin to wear makeup. By the end of four weeks the redness should fade to pink. Continuous daily use of a sunscreen with both UVA and UVB protection is essential after any peeling procedure.

Potential Risks or Side Effects

Possible complications may include infection, scarring, temporary or permanent color change in the skin and uneven pigment changes. Phenol may pose a risk for patients with a history of heart disease and any peel carries the risk of cold sores in persons who have a history of recurring fever blisters or herpes. Before undergoing any peel tell your physician if you have a history of cold sores, a tendency to scar unusually, a family history of heart problems, or have undergone radiation or numerous x-rays to the face. Darker skin types are at a higher risk for hyperpigmentation and skin discoloration.

Fees: The different treatments vary in cost according to the area treated, the individual physician and the geographic location. Generally, an AHA treatment can range from $75 to $250, whereas TCA and Phenol peel treatment can cost from $1,000 to $5,000. Typically peel treatments preformed in a medical setting are more invasive than treatments done in a salon or spa, where only superficial peels are usually offered.

"It is not sufficient to see and to know the beauty of a work. We must feel and be affected by it."

Voltaire [Francois-Marie Arouet]

LASERS AND LIGHT SOURCES

A laser is a high-energy beam of light that can selectively direct its energy into the tissue to allow the doctor greater control. In many cases, it can provide the doctor with more control over the penetration of the skin than other resurfacing treatments, such as chemical peels and microdermabrasion. These beams can be targeted to a specific point and varied in intensity and in the duration of emitted pulses. In addition to skin resurfacing, lasers can be used to treat numerous skin conditions including acne scars, unwanted hair, tattoos, discolorations and age spots. Darker skin types can be treated but the risk of pigmentation disturbances after laser treatment is higher. Different types of lasers are suited to treating specific problems. The newer techniques penetrate through to the layers beneath to boost collagen production, which gives the skin a fresher, plumper, more youthful appearance. Each is selected to treat specific skin conditions because they work slightly differently.

Ablative Lasers

Ablative laser resurfacing focus laser energy on to damaged surface layers of skin and vaporize them. This allows a fresh layer to emerge and stimulates fibroblasts. Because of the laser beam's precision, the doctor can in one session make several passes over areas that require extra attention without harm to adjacent skin. The two most frequently used deeper lasers for skin resurfacing are Carbon Dioxide CO_2 and Erbium:YAG. Brief high intensity emissions of light from the laser remove layers of damaged or wrinkled skin at precisely controlled levels of penetration. To begin, the doctor or an assistant will cleanse your face to remove oils from the skin. Antibiotic is then applied. A beam of light is passed over the skin to vapor-

LASER THERAPY
APPLICATIONS

- Acne scarring
- Active acne
- Age spots
- Birthmarks
- Hair removal
- Hemangiomas
- Hyperpigmentation
- Moles
- Port Wine Stains
- Psoriasis
- Raised scars
- Repigmentation
- Skin cancers
- Skin contraction
- Spider Veins
- Sun damage
- Tattoo removal
- Varicose Veins
- Wrinkles

ize the outer layers of damaged skin. The laser can be programmed for various levels of penetration. The doctor may choose to penetrate more deeply in some areas that need more work. As the laser works you may hear it zapping and smell smoke. Finally, an occlusive ointment or bandage will be applied to the treated area. Ablative resurfacing is normally performed under local anesthetic with intravenous sedation. The laser is passed over the area to be treated and literally evaporates the targeted areas of skin, leaving only a faint trace of smoke behind and revealing the lower layer of new, pink skin. By making more passes, the physician can avoid leaving a noticeable line of demarcation where the laser did not pass, such as at the jaw line and the area in front of the ears. The laser is passed over the face and evaporates the surface layers of the targeted areas of skin so that a new layer of pink skin is revealed. Generally, the more numerous and deep the passes of the laser, the more extensive the treatment and longer the recovery. The fairer your skin, the longer you may stay pink. These laser procedures also involve 7 to 14 days of postoperative care.

Carbon Dioxide: The Carbon Dioxide laser is considered the workhorse of laser devices. The treatment can reach the deeper wrinkles because it heats the tissues more intensely. This is a more serious treatment with a longer recovery period that can range from one to three months. When energy is delivered into the skin over a certain temperature, superficial tissues are vaporized and ablated or destroyed. CO_2 is still considered the workhorse of lasers because of its ability to cause up to 30 per cent skin shrinkage and its dramatic results on deeper wrinkles. Typically, after treatment you will be required to apply an occlusive ointment for at least a week when the epidermis regenerates.

Erbium:YAG: This technology has gained wide acceptance as the cousin to Carbon Dioxide, but without some of the side effects. The milder Erbium:YAG works well on fine lines and wrinkles, mild sun damage and scars. These lasers target the skin itself and the wavelengths are absorbed by water. Since most of our cells are predominantly water, these wavelengths are absorbed by the first cells they touch. The heat effects of the laser are scattered so that thin layers of tissue can be removed with precision while minimizing damage to surrounding skin. Techniques combining Erbium with CO2 can sometimes produce better results and speed up the long healing process. There is less risk of severe changes in color and the whitening effects. The treatment is like getting a medium depth peel and works best for mild to moderate skin damage. Long pulse Erbium:YAG lasers deliver results that fall somewhere between the CO2 and the Erbium:YAG. If needed, you can always repeat the treatment in the future.

CLASSIFICATION OF LASER DEVICES

Ablative lasers: Reserved for deeper wrinkles and creases. Ablative lasers literally remove damaged upper layers of skin, allowing a fresh layer to emerge. The most commonly used ablative lasers are the carbon dioxide (CO2) laser and the Erbium:YAG laser. Ablative lasers remove the top layer of skin. One treatment is usually all that is needed to achieve the desired results.

Non-ablative lasers: These gentler laser devices do not involve resurfacing, but rather uses the laser's heat to stimulate fibroblast production, thereby thickening the underlying collagen structure. These lasers also act as thermescent fibroblast stimulators; they heat the skin and cause the collagen to contract. Treatment is repeated monthly several times for desired results. Non-Ablative procedures are good for improving the quality, texture and tone of the skin.

Electrosurgical Resurfacing: Electrosurgical resurfacing, also called 'cold ablation' or coblation, uses a micro-electrical radio frequency to deliver a pulse of energy to the skin, removing or improving superficial to moderate skin damage. Coblation delivers electrical energy into the surface of the skin instead of heat, as lasers do. It seals blood vessels as it removes tissue and promotes skin tightening as a laser would, but by a dramatically cooler process. Electrosurgical resurfacing is applicable to most skin types and colors, without loss of skin pigmentation. It is a less expensive than many lasers and can sometimes offer faster healing; however the benefits on lines and wrinkles may not last as long.

Non-Ablative Lasers

This class of lasers does not produce a deep burn and they give a much less invasive treatment that improves skin texture and tone by stimulating new collagen in the skin to smooth it out from underneath. These treatments do not destroy outer tissue as they work their way down to stimulate collagen growth in the dermis. Each device delivers controlled energy to the skin in slightly different ways, but the process is gradual and the softening of wrinkles occurs over time as the rejuvenated skin fibers reach the skin surface. Treatments are usually repeated every four to six weeks over a six month period to maximize new collagen formation. Since non-ablative lasers often have a very long wavelength, they are relatively safe for a variety of skin types. A topical anesthetic may be all that is necessary to numb the skin for more superficial procedures. Non-ablative lasers are ideal for maintenance after more aggressive resurfacing, or as part of a total maintenance program in combination with skin care and peels or microdermabrasion treatments. Most people will see an improvement in 30 days and may continue to see improvements for up to 90 days. The newly formed collagen will then age at the normal rate and you can repeat the procedure for maintenance as needed.

Intense Pulsed Light Sources: These light sources work by creating a wound in the small blood vessels found in the dermis that causes collagen and blood vessels under the top layer to constrict. The light energy is delivered through the skin removing facial redness, erasing pigmented spots, reducing pore size and minimizing fine lines. A series of five or six photo facial treatments are given at 3-4 week intervals. There may be some minor discomfort similar to a rubber band snapping against the skin. Patients can return to work or resume their normal activities immediately after the procedure. After one or two treatments your skin will have more even tone and smoother skin. If you have rosacea and facial flushing you can expect to see a reduction in redness after each treatment. This treatment is good for fine lines particularly around the eyes and mouth shallow acne scars, age spots, broken blood vessels, large pores, and chronic facial redness. It can also be used to treat sun damaged areas on the neck, arms and chest, and hands.

Non-ablative lasers are ideal for maintenance after more aggressive resurfacing, or as part of a total maintenance program in combination with skin care and peels or microdermabrasion treatments.

Radiofrequency Waves: Devices utilizing radiofrequency waves are being evaluated for skin rejuvenation. Using radio frequency to tighten loose skin on the neck, face and body areas works by delivering deep intense heat into the skin without injury to the epidermis. The system is comprised of a radio frequency (RF) generator; a controlled modular cooling system that houses a cryogen canister and related cooling control components; and a hand-held treatment tip that couples both the cryogen cooling and the RF heating device to the treated area. One treatment may be sufficient depending on the area, but studies are underway to demonstrate the effects of multiple treatments.

PhotoDynamic Therapy: Laser-assisted photodynamic therapy (PDT) is being used as an alternative to freezing with liquid nitrogen and topical chemotherapy for brown spots called 'actinic keratoses.' The treatment works in two stages. First, a light-activated aminolevulinic acid is applied to the skin. About 14 hours later, a pulsed-dye laser light seeks out and selectively treats only the acid covered areas. PDT therapy may also be used for facial rejuvenation.

LED Technology: Photomodulation refers to using low-energy light to accelerate or inhibit cell activity. Basically, during the treatment, you would sit in front of a panel of low level light emitting diodes (LED's). Unlike laser technology that relies on high-powered coherent light to create heat energy, LED photomodulation triggers the body to convert light energy into cell energy without damaging the tissues with heat.

Post Procedure

After the skin has been treated with a laser it will be covered with either a thin film of antibiotic cream or a synthetic breathable skin to protect the newly surfaced tissue for the first five to ten days during the healing process. Redness and swelling and slight discomfort are to be expected. Regular icing can relieve some of the swelling for the first 48 hours, but you must avoid getting the area wet. Expect some redness, oozing, swelling and discomfort. If a bandage was applied after the surgery, it may be changed in a few days and removed after one week, at which time an ointment is applied. Because the bandage must remain dry, you will not be able to shower normally until it is removed. If the treated area is not bandaged, you will wash your face several times daily and apply an ointment, such as petroleum jelly. Crusting will last for 10 days after surgery, and scabs should be left alone to heal. Picking at the scabs may cause permanent scarring. You may have to drink through a straw at first for treatments around the mouth area. The healing time depends on the depth to which the laser penetrated. It may take a week or more for the skin to repair itself. The skin will turn pink, but it may take up to six months for the redness to completely fade and up to one year for normal pigmentation to return. The redness gradually lightens to pink, and then to a lighter,

A WORD ABOUT LASERS & LIGHT SOURCES

Technology changes constantly and new lasers and light sources continually come to market offering more effective and safer options. Often several devices may be used to effectively treat specific conditions. It is nearly impossible for a consumer to keep up to date with new technologies as they are introduced and to be able to evaluate which is appropriate for your particular skin type and concern. Usually, many treatments can be used in the right hands to accomplish the same goals. The best advice is to select a qualified physician you trust and let his or her recommendations guide you, rather than being persuaded by individual technologies.

more natural color. Camouflage makeup can be applied at about 10-14 days to cover up redness. Your doctor will let you know when you can use alpha hydroxy acids and retinoids acid, usually at least three to four weeks after resurfacing. Absolutely NO sun exposure will be allowed for four to eight weeks and broad spectrum sunscreen with UVA and UVB block should be worn at all times.

> *No resurfacing procedure can stop the aging process, nor is it a substitute for a face-lift. Lines and wrinkles will eventually recur.*

Duration: Laser resurfacing can be used to reduce wrinkles, scars, discoloration and imperfections in the treated area to some degree, but natural facial movements and expressions eventually cause some of the lines to reappear. Laser treatments may be repeated to maintain the desired results. No resurfacing procedure can stop the aging process, nor is it a substitute for a face-lift. Lines and wrinkles will eventually recur.

Risks or Potential Side Effects

There is a possibility of complications including infection, blisters, burns, scarring, temporary or permanent loss of sensation or pigmentation changes. Any skin resurfacing treatment carries the risk of cold sores in persons who have a history of recurring fever blisters or herpes simplex. Acne breakouts are common after resurfacing, especially if you have a previous history of acne. Milia, very small superficial cysts, may appear on the treated skin. Contact dermatitis can develop following treatment due to the use of antibiotic ointments. Adhesions may occur when treated areas of skin remain in contact with each other after the procedure and heal together, forming a small fold in the skin. This risk is decreased by ensuring that problems areas, such as the lower eyelid, are taut when the dressing is applied after the procedure. Ectropion is a rare but serious complication of laser resurfacing around the eye area. There can sometimes be a pulling down of the lower lids making it appear inverted. People of color tend to be more prone to permanent discoloration or blotchiness, hyperpigmentation or skin darkening. Sometimes a spot test may be suggested to determine if you are a good candidate for the procedure.

Fees: Different treatments vary in cost according to the area treated and the technology used. Laser treatments are usually more expensive than chemical peels and microdermabrasion largely because the technology is very pricey for doctors. Generally, full-face laser resurfacing treatments range from $2,750 to $4,200; partial face treatments cost $1,000 to $2,600.

section

V

COSMETIC DENTISTRY

If the prospect of showing your teeth in public can wipe the smile right off your face, it might be time for a state-of-the-art smile overhaul. Your teeth can really give away your age. Cosmetic and restorative dentists have the skills and tools to fill gaps, smooth chips, eliminate stains, erase cracks, and shape contours as well as making teeth whiter and brighter again. Almost any smile can be made picture- perfect these days. Although each case is unique, some new smiles can be created in just a single visit. Just as Plastic Surgeons mold soft tissues and alter the bone structure to rejuvenate the face, Cosmetic Dentists now have the ability to give you the smile you used to have or the one you wish you were born with.

Most people are not totally satisfied with their teeth, but few of us realize how simple it is to change a smile. If you're embarrassed by your teeth, you have probably trained yourself subconsciously to hide them. You may tend to talk with your lips tightly pursed or smile and laugh without showing any teeth. Cosmetics is still a relatively new branch of dentistry that marries form and function to create attractive, custom smiles that function in a state of optimum health. Before scheduling a consultation with a Cosmetic Dentist, take a few moments to study your own teeth and determine what you would most like to change.

The options in cosmetic dentistry today are virtually unlimited. Depending on the structural integrity of your teeth, the health of your gums, and your bite, crowns or orthodontics may be recommended instead of, or in addition to, veneers. In some cases, a

EVALUATING YOUR SMILE
What Dentists Look For

- When you smile normally, can you see your gum line?
- Are your two upper front teeth too wide?
- Are your two upper front teeth longer than the adjacent teeth?
- Are your upper six front teeth even in length?
- Do you have a space between your two front teeth?
- Do your front teeth protrude, stick out, and overlap?
- Do your front teeth have a crowded appearance?
- When you smile broadly, are your teeth uniform in color?
- Are your teeth stained? White, gray, brown, yellow?
- Do your fillings match the shade of your teeth?
- Are your lower six front teeth straight?
- Are your lower six front teeth even in appearance?
- When you smile widely so that the back teeth show, can you see old metallic fillings?
- Are there any signs of tooth erosion?
- When you smile broadly, do your gums show on the top teeth?
- Are your two front cuspids protruding or too long?
- Are your gums pink and healthy-looking, or red and swollen?
- Have your gums receded from the necks of the teeth?
- Does the curvature of your gum around each tooth create a half-moon shape?

chip in a front tooth, worn edges, or shallow pits or grooves in the tooth enamel can be improved with cosmetic contouring and reshaping alone, or combined with the use of veneers. Using a polishing instrument your dentist can remove small amounts of surface enamel to minimize imperfections. It is quite common for dentists to combine several techniques to achieve the best aesthetic result. For example, a typical treatment plan may include porcelain laminates placed alongside cosmetic contouring and adjoining teeth and perhaps laser bleaching for the lower arch. A skilled dentist with a trained aesthetic eye can offer you multiple scenarios to achieve your cosmetic goals within your budget. The two main cosmetic options are whitening with bleaching programs and covering-up with porcelain veneers. Because of the cost and time investment involved with extensive cosmetic dental restorations, a second or third opinion is a worthwhile investment before proceeding. If you are unhappy with your progress, it is far more difficult and costly to switch to a new dentist midstream. Another important variable to consider before embarking on elaborate dental restorations is the quality and reputation of the lab your dentist will be using.

The following chapters will illustrate the most common techniques and their variations to give you an overview of what is available.

chapter 31

"A lot of women spend $300-$400 on a dress they wear only a few times. You wear your smile your whole life."

USA Today March 26, 2003
William Dorfman, DDS,

TEETH WHITENING

Teeth whitening has become as commonplace as BOTOX® injections. Teeth lose their whiteness for a number of different reasons. As you age the outer layer of enamel on your teeth gets worn away. Eventually it reveals the darker tissue underneath, at the center of your tooth around the nerves and blood vessels. Although the fluoride in water makes teeth stronger, it can also contribute to discoloration. Some medicines, such as the antibiotic tetracycline, can also darken teeth. Some teeth just start out dark, while others become stained over time from smoking or drinking dark liquids, or from medications. Bleaching is a safe, effective means to whiten stained, discolored or dull teeth or even a single tooth. For very deep stains, only bonding or veneers can cover them up sufficiently. Porcelain veneers offer the most effective option for teeth that are discolored due to genetic, medical or environmental reasons.

ANATOMY OF A STAIN

Surface Stains: typically dark brown in color, caused by staining agents such as tannic acid, tobacco

Deposits: bacterial in origin, caused by plaque build up over time and poor oral hygiene

Structural Stains: typically show up as white blotches or brownish gray banding, often caused by tetracycline use in children or minocycline use in adults

Treatment Methods

TEETH WHITENING METHODS

- Over the Counter Bleaching Systems
- Professional Home Bleaching
- Chairside Power or Laser Bleaching
- Microabrasion
- Bonding
- Porcelain Veneers
- Crowns

Bleaching programs are a mainstay in the dentist's arsenal of beautifying treatments. At the first visit your dentist will take a complete medical history, examine your teeth and take photos and/or x-rays. Any large cavities may need to be addressed before bleaching can begin. Results will vary depending on the darkness of your teeth and the cause of the discoloration. Bleaching agents work best on yellow or brown teeth and are not as effective on gray-colored stains.

The most common element in any bleaching system is peroxide. The bleaching gel is usually hydrogen or carbamide peroxide that breaks down into oxygen molecules. The molecules go into the tiny pores of the enamel and dentin, and break up the stains that block out the light. As the stains are broken into smaller and smaller pieces, more light passes through the teeth and makes them look lighter. Stains that are accumulated over time that are yellow to slightly brown produce the best results. Teeth that are dark brown to bluish gray are the most difficult to bleach because the stain is deeply embedded in the tooth's structure. These types of stains are usually caused by medications taken during the development of the teeth. Deeper stains take a minimum of three weeks to see results and as much as six months for complete results.

Professional Home Bleaching: For home systems to be effective, the trays should be individually customized to your mouth by your dentist. Your dentist takes impressions of your teeth to create a perfectly fitted mouthpiece. This mouthpiece will hold a bleaching solution while protecting the rest of the mouth from these harsh chemicals. Contact with the teeth causes the gel to release oxygen, which begins the bleaching process. The tray can be worn overnight or for several hours each day. Depending on the bleaching gel used and the length of time it is worn, most results can be seen within three to four days. Lightly to moderately stained yellow teeth can respond well to this method. Complete results can be achieved in as little as a week or as much as several months, depending on the source and severity of the stains.

Chairside Power Bleaching: The concentration of hydrogen peroxide or carbamide peroxide in the gel is stronger for power or laser bleaching procedures. The treatment can take from one to two hours, and some people need a touch up every six months to two years, depending on personal habits. To brighten the color back up, a simple process of bleaching for one or two nights wearing the customized trays with a single syringe of bleaching gel is usually sufficient.

Laser Bleaching: Your dentist will apply a protective material to your gums and lips to protect the teeth. A special bleaching solution containing hydrogen peroxide is applied to the teeth. A high intensity light or Argon laser is directed at the teeth and activates the bleaching agent, causing the gel to release the oxygen molecules. This technique works well for a single discolored tooth. If the tooth has become dark due to trauma, but has not had a root canal, the bleaching solution is placed on the outside of the tooth. If the tooth has had a root canal, the solution can be placed on the outside as well as the inside of the tooth. Leaving a bleaching solution inside the tooth and sealing the opening is called "walking bleach". The solution inside the tooth is changed about once a week. Results take several weeks but nothing has to be worn in the mouth. Laser bleaching can take between one and two hours.

Over the Counter Bleaching Systems: Bleaching kits are available in pharmacies and supermarkets, beauty retailers, and on the Internet. These are not as effective as in office treatment and can be damaging to the gum tissue and enamel if they are too harsh. A bleaching solution is the most conservative method of whitening teeth. Whitening toothpaste is the cheapest option, but it is the least effective of all because it stays on the teeth for only a short time.

Microabrasion: A safe, effective technique to improve teeth that have a speckled appearance from chalky white spots caused by bacteria that is not sufficiently removed. The dentist carefully rubs a compound on the teeth to remove the bright white spots, so the teeth will have a more even color. These spots are difficult to treat with just bleaching. Your dentist may recommend a procedure called microabrasion. This procedure can be done by itself or in conjunction with bleaching. The microabrasion material is much like the paste used to clean and polish teeth. The paste consists of an abrasive combined with a hydrochloric acid used to "polish" out the white or brown spots. The procedure usually can be performed in one office visit and can be done without anesthesia.

Post Procedure: The amount of discomfort varies and depends on the method used. Most adults experience little, if any, discomfort. If the discomfort lasts for more than two to three days, you may need to use a gel fluoride, under your dentist's instruction, in your bleaching tray for an hour or so. Although the results of bleaching are variable, most people can get some improvement after one treatment. After any bleaching treatment

FOODS THAT STAIN TEETH

FOODS THAT STAIN TEETH	Colas, Coffee, tea, Berries (blueberries, cranberries, boysenberries, etc.), Tomato sauce, Brown gravy, Soy sauce, Red wine, Grape juice, Cherries, Balsamic vinegar, Raisins
STAIN AVOIDING TIPS	Avoid dark foods. Switch to lighter colored foods whenever possible. Drink water or rinse your mouth with water after eating or drinking. Drink darker liquids through a straw. Avoid smoking and nicotine.
FOODS THAT INTERFERE WITH THE BLEACHING PROCESS	Refined sugars, Citrus fruits and juices, Antacids, Candy, mints

avoid foods that stain for about a week because the teeth will remain very porous. Brushing well after meals, at least twice daily, and having quarterly professional cleanings will help to avoid plaque accumulation.

Risks and Limitations: Most whitening methods work to some degree and carry their own risks. Bleaching can produce side effects including increased tooth sensitivity, irritation and tenderness in the gums, tongue and other soft tissues; however, controlled bleaching does not permanently damage your teeth. Too much bleaching can make teeth brittle or too sensitive. For very sensitive teeth, periodontal disease, or teeth with worn enamel, bleaching may be discouraged. Over-bleaching may result in a translucency that may appear gray from the shadows of the mouth. With home bleaching there is a small risk of ingesting the gel administered by the dentist. If the gel is ingested it may cause nausea, vomiting or a burning sensation. The chances are relatively small since your bleaching tray will be molded to fit perfectly around your teeth.

Duration: All bleaching will regress over time, starting at around six months. You may need a touch-up with a tray method bleaching gel at home for one to two evenings to bring the white color back to the shade accomplished immediately after the initial bleaching process. Maintenance is key. The tray method is also recommended in cases where color control is critical and can be monitored by a slow and more conservative process.

Fees: Cost of the treatment ranges from and patient to patient depending on the difficulty and severity of the case. Take-home type treatments can range from $100 to $500. In-office treatments can range from $500 to $2,000 for lasers.

"The wonderful thing about veneers, is that you can do anything. You can make crooked teeth appear straight. You can make shorter teeth look longer. You can make longer teeth look shorter. You can close spaces. You can change color, size, spacing, shape and position. Veneers allow you to create an optical illusion."

"Smile Therapy", W, March 2001
Marc Lowenberg, DDS

PORCELAIN VENEERS

Porcelain veneers or laminates have been called the "gold standard" of cosmetic dentistry. The two most commonly requested treatments in cosmetic dentistry today are teeth whitening and veneers. If your goal is a true smile makeover, the most effective long term method is with beautifully customized porcelain veneers. Your natural teeth are gently shaped and thin layers of glazed porcelain are fitted on top and bonded to the tooth. This technique has several advantages over other tooth restoration procedures and is very versatile. Porcelain is an extremely durable material with a color, translucence and texture that is similar to tooth enamel. Etched porcelain provides an extremely good bond to enamel. The material is not susceptible to decay and is highly resistant to staining, losing luster or color change. If your natural teeth are discolored, you may consider whitening your teeth before veneers are applied, since extremely deep dark stains could potentially show through the thin porcelain shell.

Treatment Methods: Porcelain veneers usually require at least two appointments to be completed. The length of time of each appointment will depend on the condition of your teeth and on how many veneers you are having done. In some cases, an entire mouth makeover can be done in two visits back to back in two days.

Initial Appointment: Following the initial consultation, your teeth will be roughened and shaped to remove part of the outer tooth enamel. This provides a better surface for bonding and allows room for the placement of the thin porcelain shell. After shaping your dentist will take impressions of your teeth, which will be used to create veneers that fit your mouth precisely. Temporary veneers may be applied to protect your teeth until your customized veneers are completed.

Second Visit: Before your veneers are permanently bonded to your teeth with composite resin cement, your teeth will be thoroughly cleaned to prepare them. A dentin bonding agent is applied to hold the veneer to the tooth. At your follow-up appointment your dentist will make sure that the veneers are the ideal size and color and fit properly. Additional shaping or trimming can be done at this time, if needed.

Post Procedure: The final office visit is scheduled in order to apply the porcelain veneers to the teeth. The teeth will be cleaned and the veneers will be bonded to the teeth with bonding cement. The cement is then hardened with a blue light, which is a process called curing.

PORCELAIN VENEERS CAN BE USED TO

- Correct discolored and stained teeth
- Improve malpositioned teeth
- Fill in spaces, gaps, chips, worn, short or twisted teeth
- Broaden your entire arch of teeth
- Make teeth look bigger or longer, as needed
- Cover old porcelain bridges and crowns when the underlying structure is intact
- Close diastemas or gaps between teeth
- Lengthen and reshape teeth
- Repair chipped, broken, or misshapen teeth
- Build out teeth that are oriented inward
- Replace braces if your front teeth require only minor movement

After your teeth have been prepared and before your permanent veneers have been applied, their appearance should be fairly normal. You may have some sensitivity mainly with ice or cold liquids. During this period you should brush regularly, as your teeth will be more susceptible to staining. Regular flossing is important since swollen or bleeding gums compromise bonding the veneers on permanently. Once your veneers are permanently placed, they will feel like a natural part of your teeth.

Risks and Limitations: Veneers can be an irreversible procedure if too much tooth enamel is removed. Since the oral cavity contains bacteria and undergoes constant temperature and pressure changes, all forms of dental restorations carry some degree of uncertainty. Veneers are not entirely indestructible. To protect them from chipping, avoid biting down into hard substances and grinding your teeth. Practicing good oral hygiene and keeping the margin where the tooth and the veneer meet as clean as possible will limit decay from developing underneath the veneer. Margins will eventually need resealing. Restorations with margins above the gum line are easier to maintain than those with margins below the gum line. On occasion, people have difficulty speaking and eating immediately after having veneers placed until they get used to them.

Duration: Veneers can last from 8 – 15 years or longer with proper care.

Fees: Fees for porcelain veneers will vary depending on the difficulty of your particular case. Veneers are more expensive than conventional bonding but they also last longer. The approximate range is from $700 up to $2,500 per tooth. It is most common to have six or eight teeth on the top arch done at one stage for uniformity, since that is the typical number of teeth that show with a normal smile. The wider your smile, the more teeth you will need to have veneered to achieve an aesthetically appealing result.

Composite Bonding

Bonding, also known as composite resin bonding, is a technique used to repair chipped, cracked, or discolored teeth, to fill in gaps between teeth, protect the root of a tooth, or as an alternative to silver amalgam fillings.

LASERS IN DENTISTRY

The Millennium Nd YAG Laser is sometimes used for gum treatments to avoid more invasive periodontal surgery. Different types of laser technology can be used for many soft and hard tissue procedures in place of a scalpel including gum shaping, high-speed bonding of white fillings, and treatment of some oral lesions, gum surgery, and cosmetic contouring. The advantage of using a laser is that there is less bleeding, swelling, infection, discomfort and the need for most sutures may be eliminated.

It involves bonding a tooth-colored resin to your tooth to change its shape or repair a defect. Bonding can be used to close small gaps between front teeth and to protect exposed roots caused by gum recession, which helps reduce tooth decay and prevents sensitivity to temperature changes. The tooth-colored bonding material can also serve as an undetectable filling substance. In general, cosmetic dentists prefer porcelain laminates and veneers to bonding due to their durability and the better quality materials available. Bonding is a less expensive alternative to veneers, but it will not last as long and often does not look as natural.

AVOID BITING DOWN ON FOODS THAT CAN CAUSE CHIPS OR CRACKS
- Ice
- Pits
- Ribs
- Bones
- Hard candy and mints
- Apples
- Carrots
- Nuts
- Crusty bread
- Corn-on-the-cob
- Peanut brittle

Treatment Methods: To complete the bonding process, one or two office visits is usually all that is needed. The first visit will average about 30-60 minutes per tooth. If a second visit is required it will usually take no more than one hour for touch-up and final polishing. The cosmetic dentist begins by selecting a shade of composite resin or bonding material that is closest to the shade of your teeth. The dentist then abrades the teeth and applies a liquid that helps the bonding material adhere to the teeth. The composite resin is applied to the teeth, smoothed into the desired shape, and hardened with a high intensity light. After the resin has hardened the dentist will make the final touches and polish the tooth until it blends nicely with the other teeth. If more than one tooth is being repaired, it may take several visits to achieve the desired results.

Post Procedure: To maintain your bonded restoration professional cleanings should be done three or four times a year to remove food stains that can accumulate in microscopic spaces on the bonded surfaces of the teeth. Your hygienist should avoid using an ultrasonic scaler, which can loosen the bond, or an air abrasive spray, which can dull the polish.

Risks and Limitations: Although bonding is less expensive than porcelain laminates or crowns, it is far less durable process. Bonded surfaces are not as strong as your natural enamel or porcelain veneers and can chip and stain. For best results long term, avoid biting down with your front teeth, especially on hard or crunchy foods. Orthodontia should be completed before having bonding done. If a retainer is worn, holding wires should be Teflon-coated since stainless steel can cause discoloration with some types of bonding materials. Any contact with metals can cause chipping. Very dark stains cannot be covered well with bonding materials and some of the tooth may need to be reduced to remove stains. Gum irritation is a common side effect of bonding.

Duration: With proper care bonding can last from three to eight years before replacement is needed. You should expect to have repolishing or repair performed as necessary.

Fees: $300-$1,000 per tooth.

chapter 33

"The earliest record of crown work is from the Etruscans over 2,500 years ago. After that, crowns disappeared until the 1700s."

History of Crowns
ADA Dental Minute
Dr. Maria Lopez Howell
© 2002

BRIDGES & CROWNS

Crowns and bridges are restorative techniques that repair damaged or missing teeth while improving function and appearance. The use of crowns and bridges also avoids shifting teeth that can happen after a tooth is lost. Like crowns, bridges are also being used less often, as implants are becoming a very popular means of replacing one or more lost teeth. A bridge is recommended when there is a missing tooth. A crown or a bridge may be the best and most cost efficient method of restoring a functional, attractive smile after tooth damage. Bridges are one method to fill a gap created by missing teeth. A bridge is made up of two crowns for the teeth on either side of the gap and a false tooth in between. Natural teeth, dental implants, or a combination of both can be used to support the bridge.

Crowns

Crowns are coverings that fit over teeth that are chipped, fractured, malformed, malpositioned or discolored. They are used to restore the tooth to its normal shape and size, while both strengthening and improving its appearance. Crowns can be made from several different kinds of materials depending on location, esthetics, and cost. The loss of a tooth or teeth changes your bite and puts stress on surrounding teeth to compensate for the lost tooth. Your dentist may suggest replacing the missing tooth with an artificial tooth connected between two crowns which are permanently cemented or bonded on the adjacent teeth. A crown is usually reserved for teeth that are beyond repair with less invasive methods like filling, inlay or onlay. Damage due to decay, accident, wear or grinding can be repaired with crowns. More conservative techniques, such as veneers, inlays, onlays, bonding, and bleaching, have replaced some of the instances when crowns were used in the past. Depending on the extent of the decay or damage, your dentist may perform a root canal before placing a crown on the tooth. In this case, your dentist may need to build a foundation for the crown after the root canal has been performed, also known as a "post-and-core" foundation. Before the crown can be placed on the tooth, the tooth must be filed down to make room for it. Then an impression of the tooth and the surrounding teeth will be made. While the crown is being created a temporary acrylic crown will be placed on the tooth. When the permanent crowns are ready the temporary crowns are replaced during a separate visit.

Treatment Methods: At the initial consultation your dentist will determine the cause of your tooth problems. If a tooth is damaged, fractured, or decayed beyond repair, a crown may be suggested. If a tooth needs to be extracted, or has already been removed, a bridge may be the solution. An important deciding factor as to whether a crown or bridge is needed is the material the laboratory will use to make the appliance. The replacement tooth can be made from different types of material such as a metal base covered with a layer of tooth-colored material that is often porcelain, or all porcelain. Metal restorations, such as gold crowns, are usually only used when the tooth is not visible. Porcelain bonded to metal crowns are more aesthetically pleasing than metal alone, although the metal layer reduces the translucency of the crown. The resulting crown is very strong but the tooth must be reduced slightly more to support this type of restoration. A final choice is full porcelain, which can be indistinguishable from

TYPES OF BRIDGES

Traditional bridge: This type of bridge consists of two crowns for the teeth on either side of the gap, with a false tooth in between. Traditional bridges are the most commonly used type of bridge and are made of ceramic or porcelain fused to metal (PFM).

Cantilever bridge: This type of bridge is used when there are teeth on only one side of the gap in the mouth.

Maryland bonded bridge: This type of bridge is made up of plastic teeth and gums supported by a metal framework.

a natural tooth, but is slightly less durable.

When deciding between a bridge and an implant, the teeth flanking the bridge may need to be reduced in order to receive the bridge structure. These alterations will not be necessary if the missing tooth is replaced with an implant. Your dentist will begin bridgework by filing down the teeth to accommodate the crowns. Impressions of the teeth will be taken which will be used to create the crowns. Once the crowns are finished, artificial teeth will be bonded to them. When the bridge is ready a return visit will be necessary to place it on the teeth.

The procedures for making and fitting a crown or a bridge are very similar. Both require at least two trips to the dentist's office:

Initial Visit: During the first trip the teeth that will be crowned will be reduced by one or two millimeters to support the crown structure. If damage is the reason for the crown, that is the part that is removed. The reduction process leaves a thimble shape that will receive the crown or crown ends of the bridge. An impression is made of the reduced teeth and a temporary crown or bridge is put in place to function while the final bridge or crown is being made. The laboratory uses the impression to custom make the final restoration. The crown or crowns of a bridge should be made to fit exactly to avoid decay and provide good function of the artificial teeth. The first visit will take about one hour or longer.

Second Visit: The temporary crown or bridge is removed, the area cleaned, and the final crown or bridge is cemented or bonded into place. Teeth can be lightened or whitened to any desired shade. If a custom shade is necessary due to various shades in the tooth, the dentist may request you visit the lab for a better match. The second visit is slightly shorter than the first and will take about forty-five minutes or longer if adjustments need to be made in the fit.

Post Procedure: Local anesthesia is used to minimize discomfort during your treatment sessions. A loosening of the temporary crown may occur between visits. If this should happen, you will be instructed to place the crown back on your tooth immediately and call your dentist's office to have the temporary crown refitted. It is important to act quickly as the surrounding teeth might move, which can affect the final restoration. It is not unusual for the teeth receiving the new crowns to be sensitive to extreme temperatures for several days following the treatment. With bridges or crowns the teeth feel back to normal within a day or two in most cases. Further adjustments may be needed with the crown or bridge placement.

When deciding between a bridge and an implant, the teeth flanking the bridge may need to be reduced in order to receive the bridge structure.

Risks and Limitations: With crowning the original tooth form is altered, which could potentially affect the nerve. As with your original smile, care must be taken to avoid tooth fractures. The placement of any restorative fixture in the mouth brings a risk of breakage. Bridges can be great traps for food, so it is critical to brush, floss, and have regular professional cleanings and fluoride treatments after it has been placed in the mouth. A diet that reduces intake of refined sugars will prevent the cement that helps hold the crowns in place from washing away due to decay. As the false tooth and the crown are a single, solid piece, it is not possible to floss between them. You will need to use a floss threader to go under the false tooth and keep the gum healthy. Depending on the materials used to manufacture the fixture, there is a greater or lesser risk of breakage.

Duration: Crowns offer the longest life of any restoration. With meticulous care, crowns and bridges last 5 - 15 years or longer. If any damage occurs to the structure of the crown or bridge an immediate trip to the dentist is recommended to avoid further damage due to the weakened structure. The life expectancy of a crown or bridge is related to fractures, problems with tissue and the potential danger of decay.

Fees: The average cost of a single fixed bridge depends on the number of teeth or units you are replacing. Bridges usually cost $600-$1,500 per unit, depending on the difficulty of your case and the material used. The average cost of a single crown is $600-$2,500. Prices may vary depending on the difficulty of your case, material of the crown used and the location of the laboratory. The cost of dental crowns depends on the type of crown used and the number of crowns placed in the mouth.

chapter 34

Beauty is power; a smile is its sword.

Charles Reade 1814-1884,
British Novelist, Dramatist

DENTAL IMPLANTS

Dental implants can be a multi-staged process involving one or several dental specialists. Implants are basically anchors that permanently hold replacement teeth. They are used to deliver artificial teeth that can be used to replace missing or decaying teeth and provide additional support combined with bridges, dentures and crowns. Replacing a lost tooth is vital to maintaining the function of the surrounding teeth. It helps avoid tooth migration, loss of structure and loss of bone from the jaw. Implants reduce the impact of the lost tooth on surrounding teeth. Traditional bridge structures often require reduction of the two adjacent teeth to hold the bridge in place with crowns. Implants are considered the best way to surgically restore a natural tooth to its original condition, and they can be an ideal alternative to a bridge if only one or a few teeth need to be replaced. Bridges attach artificial teeth to existing teeth, but implants attach directly to the jawbone or under the tissues of the gums. Implants are the most permanent method of replacing missing teeth. Their main advantages are that they look and feel natural and fit very securely, which allows for better chewing ability and eliminates the embarrassment of dentures. There are several different types of implants, but the most popular are metal screws surgically placed into the jaw bones. Implants are considered permanent and stable since they don't rely on other teeth for support, as with other dental appliances.

Types of Dental Implants

Root-form implant: This is the most common type of dental implant, also called endosseous or endosteal implant because the implant is placed in the bone. Root-form implants are made of titanium and are similar in appearance to screws, nails or cones.

Sub-periosteal implant: These types of implants are not placed in the bone. They ride above the bone but beneath the gum. A CAT scan is commonly used to obtain a model of the bone structure and then the implant fixture is molded to precisely fit the bone model.

Plate-form implant: This type of implant is a rectangle of metal with either one or two metal prongs on one side. Plate - form implants are placed vertically in the jaw so that the prongs stick up into the mouth and provide a place for the artificial tooth to be placed.

Ramus-frame implant: These are commonly used when there is a thin lower jawbone. Ramus-frame implants are placed in the jaw at the back of the mouth and near the chin. Dentures are then made to fit on the thin metal bar that is visible above the gum tissue.

QUESTIONS TO ASK ABOUT DENTAL IMPLANTS

- What are the expected benefits of this procedure and what kind of improvement can I expect?
- What are the risks of this procedure in my case?
- What is your estimated cost of the procedure and what is included in your fee?
- How many of these procedures have you done?
- Is there an alternative treatment that I should consider?
- How long will the procedure take and how many appointments will be necessary?
- Will you repeat or correct procedures if the outcome does not meet agreed upon goals? The dentist should provide you with his/her policy on revisions.
- What kind of longevity can I expect?
- May I look at before and after photos of recent patients you have performed this procedure on?
- What should I expect after the procedure?

Bone Grafting: This involves moving bone from one place in the body to another to enlarge the bone structure at the implant site. Sometimes a graft from a donor or artificial bone can also be used.

Treatment Methods: The procedure is usually done in two or more

IMPLANT CHARACTERISTICS

ROOT-FORM IMPLANT	
	• Most common type of dental implant also called endosseous or endosteal implant • Implant placed in the bone made in titanium • Looks like a screw, nail or cone
SUB-PERIOSTEAL IMPLANT	
	• Placed above the bone but beneath the gum
PLATE-FORM IMPLANT	
	• Rectangle of metal with one or two metal prongs on one side • Placed vertically in the jaw • Prongs provide a place for the artificial tooth to be placed
RAMUS-FRAME IMPLANT	
	• Commonly used when there is a thin lower jawbone • Placed in the jaw at the back of the mouth and near the chin • Dentures are made to fit on the thin metal
BONE GRAFTING	
	• Involves moving bone from one place in the body to another • Its aim is to enlarge the bone structure at the implant site • A graft from a donor or artificial bone can be also used

stages. The initial surgery to position an anchor in the jaw to allow the bone to grow around may be followed by a second procedure to place a post-like fixture used to connect the anchor to the artificial teeth.

Because bone heals slowly, treatment with implants can often take longer than bridges or dentures. Implants in the upper jaw will take approximately six months; implants in the lower jaw will take approximately three months.

Initial Stage: At your first appointment, the dentist will examine your teeth to determine whether implants are the best solution and what type of implant is needed. X-rays will be needed to discover the state of the jawbone, particularly if the teeth have been missing for some time. Under local anesthesia, the first step is the exposure of the bone where the implant is to be made. An incision is made in the gums, exposing the bone in the jaw, and a hole is made where the dental implant is located. Tiny titanium posts are threaded like a screw into your jawbone. The implant is then placed into the bone and the gums are closed with stitches. The bone then grows around these posts, anchoring them. If there isn't enough bone, a separate surgical procedure to add bone may be needed. Bone grafting is typically done four to eight months before the implant procedure, to allow the graft a chance to heal before it is disturbed with the implant process. After placement of the implant a cover screw is put in and the wound is closed with stitches. The bone is given time to grow and fuse around it. Because bone heals slowly, treatment with implants can often take longer than bridges or dentures. Implants in the upper jaw will take approximately six months; implants in the lower jaw will take approximately three months.

Stage Two: After the jaw heals and the bone has grown around the implant, a process known as osseointegration, the second procedure is performed. Permanent porcelain bridges or individual teeth are screwed or cemented onto the titanium posts. The artificial tooth is then added, depending on the type of dental implant used, and any necessary bridges or dentures can be fitted to the teeth.

Risks and Limitations: The primary consideration for the suitability of dental implants is the amount and condition of the bone in the area where the implant is to be placed. With the loss of a tooth, the area of the jaw without the tooth naturally undergoes resorption, or a thinning, of the bone in that area. Location of the implant can also predict the risk of failure. The less healthy bone available at the site to place the implant, the greater chance of implant failure. For implants placed within the bone, most failures occur within the first year and then occur at a rate of less than one percent per year thereafter. Implants in the back upper jaw fail most often, followed by the front upper jaw, the back lower jaw, and the most success is seen in implants of the front lower jaw. Most failed implants can be replaced with a second attempt. To be a candidate for implant surgery you must also have healthy gums. In addition to practicing good oral hygiene, you will need regular check-ups to maintain your implants. If you have sensitive teeth caused by receding gums, your dentist may suggest using special toothpaste for a few months.

Duration: Implants may last between fifteen and twenty-five years. Five to ten percent of implants fail on the first attempt. Poor hygiene can result in chronic swelling of gum tissue and is often a major contributor to implant failure. You will need to see your dentist about four times a year to maintain good hygiene and the health of the implants.

Fees: Implants can be very costly, particularly if several are needed to restore the teeth lost. Each surgical step has separate costs, as do the fixtures and materials themselves. Single teeth run between about $1,500 to about $4,000 with multiple implants costing more. Full sets of implanted teeth can run as high as $30,000. Most dental plans do not cover the cost of implants.

"More people are getting braces than ever before—even adults. In fact, of 5 million orthodontic patients in the United States and Canada, one in five is an adult, according to the American Association of Orthodontics (AAO)."

New Faces of Braces Younger—and Much Older—Patients are Benefiting From Orthodontics
By La Rue V. Baber Staff Writer
Los Angeles Daily News, Sunday, October 27, 2002

ORTHODONTICS

Orthodontics deals with straightening teeth and correcting irregular bites known as malocclusion through the use of corrective appliances, including braces and retainers. Typically an orthodontist will work with you to develop a specific treatment plan outlining the type of appliance required and the expected length of time until therapy will be completed. Braces are used to correct crowded and overlapping teeth in children, teens, as well as adults.

Some people may have had orthodontic treatment when they were young, but did not wear their retainers until they stopped growing. The result may be that their teeth are slightly crooked as adults. As much as one quarter of all orthodontic treatment is being done for adults today. When you are growing your jaw is like clay; if your mouth is too small for your teeth, the orthodontist can stretch your mouth so everything fits. Once you stop growing, and after your jaw hardens, it becomes more difficult to stretch your jaw. Some people have their jaw enlarged surgically, although adults tend to choose to have their teeth straightened, but not have their jaw enlarged. The orthodontist may then have to remove some teeth to make everything fit. The process may be slightly more uncomfortable when you are older. There is no age limit, although orthodontic treatment goes slower when you are older, so it may take longer to get the results you want. The orthodontist can still move your teeth, but your teeth have to move more slowly to let your mouth heal between tightening appointments. Not all adults are candidates for orthodontia. For example, some adults have gums which have receded too much, or have shallow roots from years of abuse. In these cases, veneers are often used instead of orthodontia.

Treatment Method

There are two phases to most orthodontic treatment:

- Active phase: use of braces to move the teeth into their new position
- Retention phase: the use of a retainer to keep the teeth in place

Braces: Braces work to move the teeth by applying continuous pressure in a specific direction. This pressure is adjusted many times over the course of the treatment, which can last anywhere from one to three years, and sometimes longer. Braces consist of brackets, which are applied to the teeth with a bonding agent, and arch wires, which are threaded through the brackets and act as a track to guide the teeth to their new position. When an orthodontist puts in your braces your mouth will be tender for about a week. As the tenderness goes away, you will hardly notice your braces except when they are tightened. When a teenager gets braces, the orthodontist is usually moving teeth that have come in fairly recently, so they are easier to move. As you get older, your teeth get anchored to your jaw with little filaments and the orthodontist needs to loosen those filaments before your teeth will move. The filaments will tighten again once your orthodontic treatment is completed.

Retainers: A retainer is an orthodontic appliance made of plastic and stainless steel wire that is used to hold the teeth in place after braces have been removed, while the surrounding bone and gums adjust around them. The length of time that the retainer must be worn will vary, but most teenagers will be advised to wear their retainer until their early twenties.

Choices in Appliances

Modern braces are smaller and more comfortable than the braces of yesteryear. They are designed to have a low profile design, which is less irritating to the lips. They also have special contours to make the orthodontic treatment less painful and go faster. Lingual braces placed behind the teeth may also be used as an alternative or in combination with more traditional treatment.

Damon Bracket: This "sliding-door" technology is known as "self-ligation" that allows the wire to slide back and forth within the bracket. This creates less friction and results in a more comfortable fit. Damon brackets cut down on the treatment time and the number of adjustments that need to be performed.

Ceramic Bracket: Ceramic brackets are translucent, so they blend in with your natural tooth color. This means that unlike traditional stainless steel braces, they are far less conspicuous. Coated white wire can be used to make them even less noticeable. These brackets are designed not to stain or discolor over long periods of time. They also come in a series of fashion colors and styles from gold to bright pink.

Invisible Braces: Invisalign®, also known as invisible braces, is an orthodontic system that works to straighten the teeth through the use of a series of clear plastic molds called aligners. The Invisalign® computer imaging system creates the aligners by simulating the stages the teeth will go through until they reach their final position. The number of aligners used will depend on each individual case, but the average is between 18 and 30. Each removable aligner is worn for two weeks 24 hours a day, except during meals, and then the next aligner is used. This process is repeated until the teeth are in the desired position. The entire treatment takes the same amount of time as traditional braces.

Post Procedure: Special care must be taken to maintain the orthodontic device and insure good oral hygiene. Retainers frequently have to be worn at night for many years, at least a few nights a week, possibly indefinitely, to maintain tooth alignment. A water-powered cleaning device is also helpful if used daily.

Risks and Limitations: The most obvious disadvantage of orthodontic treatment is that is it a time-intensive process and cannot be rushed. The appliances can be uncomfortable until you get used to wearing them continuously. New models continue to be more inconspicuous so they can be worn without feeling self-conscious. It is possible that your teeth may return to their original position if retainers are not worn sufficiently.

Duration: Orthodontic treatment may take 6 months to 2 years or longer to complete. The results are considered permanent in most cases.

Fees: Braces can be stainless steel, plastic or ceramic. Stainless steel is the most common. The cost of braces varies depending on the type of braces used and the length of treatment, but ranges between $2,000 and $7,500. Invisible braces are often more costly than traditional orthodontic treatment. Orthodontics may be less expensive than laminating, crowning or bonding, depending on the number of teeth involved. In certain cases, orthodontic treatment may be covered by your dental insurance or you may be able to purchase a special rider to cover medically necessary orthodontia.

section

VI

APPENDICES

Many of the following appendices have been referred to in the text. Others were added to provide additional information to help you make the most informed decision when choosing a cosmetic doctor or dentist.

Appendix A

STATE MEDICAL BOARDS

Alabama State Board of Medical Examiners
P.O. Box 946
Montgomery, AL 36101-0946
(street address: 848 Washington Ave., 36104)
(334) 242-4116 / Fax: (334) 242-4155
(800) 227-2606
www.albme.org

Alaska State Medical Board
3601 C Street, Suite 722
Anchorage, AK 99503-5986
(907) 269-8163 / Fax: (907) 269-8196
www.dced.state.ak. us/occ/pmed.htm

Arizona Board of Medical Examiners
9545 East Doubletree Ranch Road
Scottsdale, AZ 85258
(480) 551-2700 / Fax: (480) 551-2701
www.bomex.org

Arizona Board of Osteopathic Examiners in Medicine and Surgery
9535 East Doubletree Ranch Road
Scottsdale, AZ 85258-5539
(480) 657-7703 / Fax: (480) 657-7715
www.azosteoboard.org

Arkansas State Medical Board
2100 Riverfront Dr., Suite 200
Little Rock, AR 72202-1793
(501) 296-1802 / Fax: (501) 296-1805
www.armedicalboard.org

Medical Board of California
1426 Howe Ave., Suite 54
Sacramento, CA 95825-3236
(916) 263-2389 / Fax: (916) 263-2387
(800) 633-2322
www.medbd.ca.gov

Osteopathic Medical Board of California
2720 Gateway Oaks Dr., Suite 350
Sacramento, CA 95833-3500
(916) 263-3100 / Fax: (916) 263-3117
www.dca.ca.gov/osteopathic

Colorado Board of Medical Examiners
1560 Broadway, Suite 1300
Denver, CO 80202-5140
(303) 894-7690 / Fax: (303) 894-7692
www.dora.state.co.us/me dical

Connecticut Medical Examining Board
P.O. Box 340308
Hartford, CT 06134-0308
(street address: 410 Capitol Ave. MS13PHO)
(860) 509-7648 / Fax: (860) 509-7553
Licensing Information,(860) 509-7563

Delaware Board of Medical Practice
P.O. Box 1401
Dover, DE 19903
(street address: 861 Silver Lake Blvd., Cannon Building, Suite 203, 19904)
(302) 739-4522 / Fax: (302) 739-2711
www.state.de.us /license/28/index.htm

District of Columbia Board of Medicine
825 North Capital Street, NE, 2nd Floor
Washington, DC 20002
(202) 442-9200 / Fax: (202) 442-9431
www.dchealth.dc.gov

Florida Board of Medicine
4052 Bald Cypress Way, BIN #C03
Tallahassee, FL 32399-1753
(850) 245-4131 / Fax: (850) 488-9325
www.doh.state.fl.us

Florida Board of Osteopathic Medicine
4052 Bald Cypress Way, BIN C06
Tallahassee, FL 32399
(street address: Northwood Centre, 1940 N. Monroe St., 32399-0757)
(850) 488-0595 / Fax: (850) 487-9874
www.doh.state.fl.us

Georgia Composite State Board of Medical Examiners
2 Peachtree Street, NW, 6th Floor
Atlanta, GA 30303-3465
(404) 656-3913 / Fax: (404) 656-9723
www.medicalboard.state. ga.us

Hawaii Board of Medical Examiners
Dept. of Commerce & Consumer Affairs
P.O. Box 3469
Honolulu, HI 96801
(street address: 1010 Richards St., 96813)
(808) 586-3000 / Fax: (808) 586-2874
www.state.hi.us

Idaho State Board of Medicine
Statehouse mail
P.O. Box 83720
Boise, ID 83720-0058
(street address: 1755 Westgate Drive, Suite 140, 83704)
(208) 327-7000 / Fax: (208) 327-7005
www.bom.state.id.us

Illinois Department of Professional Regulation
(Discipline)
James R. Thompson Center
100 W. Randolph St., 9-300
Chicago, IL 60601
(312) 814-4500 / Fax: (312) 814-1837

(Licensure)
320 W. Washington St., 3rd Floor
Springfield, IL 62786
(217) 785-0800 / Fax: (217) 524-2169
www.dpr.state.il.us

Indiana Health Professions Bureau
402 W. Washington St., Room 041
Indianapolis, IN 46204
(317) 232-2960 / Fax: (317) 233-4236
www.ai.org/hpb

Iowa State Board of Medical Examiners
400 Southwest Eighth Street, Suite C
Des Moines, IA 50309-4686
(515) 281-5171 / Fax: (515) 242-5908
www.docboard.org/ia/ia_home.htm

Kansas Board of Healing Arts
235 SW Topeka Blvd.
Topeka, KS 66603-3068
(785) 296-7413 / Fax: (785) 296-0852
www.ink.org/public/boha

Kentucky Board of Medical Licensure
Hurstbourne Office Park
310 Whittington Parkway, Suite 1B
Louisville, KY 40222-4916
(502) 429-8046 / Fax: (502) 429-9923
www.state.ky.us/agencies/kbml

Louisiana State Board of Medical Examiners
P.O. Box 30250
New Orleans, LA 70190-0250
(street address: 630 Camp St., 70130)
(504) 568-6820 / Fax: (504) 568-8893
www.lsbme.org

Maine Board of Licensure in Medicine
137 State House Station (U.S. mail)
2 Bangor Street, 2nd Floor (delivery service)
Augusta, ME 04333
(207) 287-3601 / Fax: (207) 287-6590
www.docboard.org/me/me_home.htm

Maine Board of Osteopathic Licensure
142 State House Station
Augusta, ME 04333-0142
(207) 287-2480 / Fax: (207) 287-3015
www.docboard.org/me-osteo

Maryland Board of Physician Quality Assurance
P.O. Box 2571
Baltimore, MD 21215-0095
(street address: 4201 Patterson Ave., third floor, 21215)
(410) 764-4777 / Fax: (410) 358-2252
(800) 492-6836
pqa.state.md.us

Massachusetts Board of Registration in Medicine
10 West St., 3rd Floor
Boston, MA 02111
(617) 727-3086 / Fax: (617) 451-9568
(800) 377-0550
www.massmedboard.org

Michigan Board of Medicine
P.O. Box 30670
Lansing, MI 48909-7518
(street address: 611 W. Ottawa St, 1st floor, 48933
(517) 373-6873 / Fax: (517) 373-2179
www.michigan.gov/cis

Michigan Board of Osteopathic Medicine and Surgery
P.O. Box 30670
Lansing, MI 48909-7518
(street address: 611 W. Ottawa St, 1st floor, 48933
(517) 373-6873 / Fax: (517) 373-2179
www.cis.state.mi.us/bhser

Minnesota Board of Medical Practice
University Park Plaza
2829 University Ave. SE, Suite 400
Minneapolis, MN 55414-3246
(612) 617-2130 / Fax: (612) 617-2166
Hearing impaired (800) 627-3529
www.bmp.state.mn.us

Mississippi State Board of Medical Licensure
1867 Crane Ridge Drive, Suite 200B
Jackson, MS 39216
(601) 987-3079 / Fax: (601) 987-4159
www.msbml.state.ms.us

Missouri State Board of Registration for the Healing Arts
P.O. Box 4
Jefferson City, MO 65102
(street address: 3605 Missouri Blvd., 65109)
(573) 751-0098 / Fax: (573) 751-3166
www.ecodev.state.mo.us/pr/healarts

Montana Board of Medical Examiners
P.O. Box 200513
Helena, MT 59620-0513
(street address: 301 S. Park Ave., 4th floor)
(406) 841-2361 / Fax: (406) 841-2363
www.discoveringmontana.com

Nebraska Health and Human Services, Regulation and Licensure
Credentialing Division
P.O. Box 94986
Lincoln, NE 68509-4986
(street address: 301 Centennial Mall South, 68508)
(402) 471-2118 / Fax: (402) 471-3577
www.hhs.state.ne.us

Nevada State Board of Medical Examiners
P.O. Box 7238
Reno, NV 89510
(street address: 1105 Terminal Way, Suite 301, 89502)
(775) 688-2559 / Fax: (775) 688-2321
www.state.nv.us/medical

Nevada State Board of Osteopathic Medicine
2860 E. Flamingo Rd., Suite G
Las Vegas, NV 89121
(702) 732-2147 / Fax: (702) 732-2079
www.osteo.state.nv.us

New Hampshire Board of Medicine
2 Industrial Park Drive, Suite 8
Concord, NH 03301-8520
(603) 271-1203 / Fax: (603) 271-6702
Complaints (800) 780-4757
www.state.nh.us/medicine

New Jersey State Board of Medical Examiners
P.O. Box 183
Trenton, NJ 08625
(street address: 140 E. Front Street, 2nd Floor)
(609) 826-7100 / Fax: (609) 826-7117
www.state.nj.us

New Mexico State Board of Medical Examiners
Lamy Building, 2nd Floor
491 Old Santa Fe Trail
Santa Fe, NM 87501
(505) 827-5022 / Fax: (505) 827-7377
www.state.nm.us/nmbme

New Mexico Board of Osteopathic Medical Examiners
P.O. Box 25101
Santa Fe, NM 87504
(street address: 2055 S. Pacheco, Suite 400)
(505) 476-7120 / Fax: (505) 476-7095
www.nmoma.org

New York State Board for Medicine (Licensure)
89 Washington Avenue, 2nd Floor, West Wing
Albany, NY 12234-1000
(518) 474-3817 Ext. 560 / Fax: (518) 486-4846
www.op.nysed.gov

New York State Board for Professional Medical Conduct (Discipline)
New York State Dept. of Health
Office of Professional Medical Conduct
433 River St., Suite 303
Troy, NY 12180
(518) 402-0855 / Fax: (518) 402-0866
www.health.state.ny.us/

North Carolina Medical Board
P.O. Box 20007
Raleigh, NC 27619-0007
(street address: 1201 Front Street, 27609)
(919) 326-1100 / Fax: (919) 326-1130
www.ncmedboard.org

North Dakota State Board of Medical Examiners
City Center Plaza
418 E. Broadway, Suite 12
Bismarck, ND 58501
(701) 328-6500 / Fax: (701) 328-6505
www.ndbomex.com

State Medical Board of Ohio
77 S. High St., 17th Floor
Columbus, OH 43266-0315 (for Fed Ex delivery use zip 43215)
(614) 466-3934 / Fax: (614) 728-5946
(800) 554-7717
www.state.oh.us/med/

Oklahoma State Board of Medical Licensure and Supervision
P.O. Box 18256
Oklahoma City, OK 73154-0256
(street address: 5104 N. Francis, Suite C, 73118)
(405) 848-6841 / Fax: (405) 848-8240
(800) 381-4519
www.osbmls.state.ok.us

Oklahoma State Board of Osteopathic Examiners
4848 N. Lincoln Blvd, Suite 100
Oklahoma City, OK 73105-3321
(405) 528-8625 / Fax: (405) 557-0653
www.docboard.org/ok.ok.htm

Oregon Board of Medical Examiners
620 Crown Plaza
1500 SW First Avenue
Portland, OR 97201-5826
(503) 229-5770 / Fax: (503) 229-6543
www.bme.state.or.us

Pennsylvania State Board of Medicine
P.O. Box 2649
Harrisburg, PA 17105-2649
street address: 124 Pine Street, 17101
(717) 787-2381 / Fax: (717) 787-7769
www.dos.state.pa.us

Pennsylvania State Board of Osteopathic Medicine
P.O. Box 2649
Harrisburg, PA 17105-2649
(street address: 124 Pine St., 17101)
(717) 783-4858 / Fax: (717) 787-7769
www.dos.state.pa.us

Board of Medical Examiners of Puerto Rico
P.O. Box 13969
San Juan, PR 00908
(street address: Kennedy Avenue, ILA Building, Hogar del Obrero
Portuario, Piso 8, Puerto Nuevo, 00920)
(787) 782-8989 / Fax: (787) 782-8733

Rhode Island Board of Medical Licensure and Discipline
Dept. of Health
Cannon Building, Room 205
Three Capitol Hill
Providence, RI 02908-5097
(401) 222-3855 / Fax: (401) 222-2158
www.docboard.org/ri/mai n.htm

South Carolina Department of Labor, Licensing and Regulation
Board of Medical Examiners
P.O. Box 11289
Columbia, SC 29211-1289
(street address: 110 Centerview Drive, Suite 202, 29210)
(803) 896-4500 / Fax: (803) 896-4515
www.llr.state.sc.us/ pol/medical

South Dakota State Board of Medical and Osteopathic Examiners
1323 S. Minnesota Ave.
Sioux Falls, SD 57105
(605) 334-8343 / Fax: (605) 336-0270
www.state.sd.us/dcr/medi cal

Tennessee Board of Medical Examiners
1st Floor, Cordell Hull Building
425 5th Ave. North
Nashville, TN 37247-1010
(615) 532-3202 / Fax: (615) 253-4484
www.state.tn.us/health

Tennessee Board of Osteopathic Examiners
425 5th Ave. North
1st Floor, Cordell Hull Building
Nashville, TN 37247-1010 (37219 Fed Ex zip code)
(615) 532-3202 / Fax: (615) 253-4484
(888) 310-4650
www.state.tn.us/health

Texas State Board of Medical Examiners
P.O. Box 2018
Austin, TX 78768-2018
(street address: 333 Guadalupe, Tower 3, Suite 630, 78701
(512) 305-7010 / Fax: (512) 305-7008
Disciplinary Hotline (800) 248-4062
Consumer Complaint Hotline (800) 201-9353
www.tsbme.state.tx.us

Utah Department of Commerce
Div. of Occupational & Professional Licensure
P.O. Box 146741
Salt Lake City, UT 84114-6741
(street address: Hebert M. Wells Building, 4th Floor, 160 E 300 South, 84102)
(801) 530-6628 / Fax: (801) 530-6511
www.commerce.state.ut.us or http://dopl.utah.gov

Utah Department of Commerce
Div. of Occupational & Professional Licensure
Board of Osteopathic Medicine
P.O. Box 146741
Salt Lake City, UT 84114-6741
(street address: Hebert M. Wells Building, 4th Floor, 160 E 300 South, 84102)
(801) 530-6628 / Fax: (801) 530-6511
www.commerce.state.ut.us

Vermont Board of Medical Practice
109 State St.
Montpelier, VT 05609-1106
(802) 828-2673 / Fax: (802) 828-5450
www.docboard.org/vt/ vermont.htm

Vermont Board of Osteopathic Physicians and Surgeons
26 Terrace Street, Drawer 09
Montpelier, VT 05609-1106
(802) 828-2373 / Fax: (802) 828-2465
www.healthyvermonters.info/bpm/bpm.shtml

Virginia Board of Medicine
6606 W. Broad St., 4th Floor
Richmond, VA 23230-1717
(804) 662-9908 / Fax: (804) 662-9517
www.dhp.state.va.us/

Washington Medical Quality Assurance Commission
P.O. Box 47866
Olympia, WA 98504-7866
(street address: 1300 SE Quince Street, 98501)
(360) 236-4888 / Fax: (360) 586-4573
www.doh.wa.gov

Washington State Board of Osteopathic Medicine and Surgery
P.O Box 47870
Olympia, WA 98504-7866
(street address: 1300 SE Quince Street, 98501)
(360) 236-4943 / Fax: (360) 586-0745
www.doh.wa.gov

West Virginia Board of Medicine
101 Dee Drive
Charleston, WV 25311
(304) 558-2921 / Fax: (304) 558-2084
www.wvdhhr.org/wvbom

West Virginia Board of Osteopathy
334 Penco Rd.
Weirton, WV 26062
(304) 723-4638 / Fax: (304) 723-2877
www.state.wv.us/bdosteo/

Wisconsin Medical Examining Board
Dept. of Regulation & Licensing
P.O. Box 8935
Madison, WI 53708-8935
(street address: 1400 E. Washington Ave., 53703)
(608) 266-2112 / Fax: (608) 267-0644
badger.state.wi.us

Wyoming Board of Medicine
211 W. 19th St., Colony Bldg., 2nd floor
Cheyenne, WY 82002
(307) 778-7053 / Fax: (307) 778-2069
wyomedboard.state.wy.us

Appendix B

SELF-DESIGNATED
MEDICAL SPECIALTIES

This list of self-designated medical specialty groups was obtained from the American Board of Medical Specialties. However, it is important to point out that these groups are not recognized by the ABMS, the governing board for the twenty-four recognized medical specialty boards.

The organizations listed below range from highly organized groups that are attempting to formalize training and certification in their field to informal groups interested in a particular aspect of medicine.

If you wish to obtain information from any of these groups you will have to do some detective work. Because so many are informal, the location, phone and mailing addresses change frequently, depending upon the person who is functioning as secretary or administrator.

The best way to track down one of these groups is to consult the doctor listings to find a doctor who has expressed a special interest in that field, and call his or her office. You might also call a nearby academic health center in the area to see if they have a faculty or staff member known to be involved in that particular medical interest. If that fails, take the same approach with your community hospital.

A

Abdominal Surgeons
Acupuncture Medicine
Addiction Medicine
Addictionology
Adolescent Psychiatry
Aesthetic Plastic Surgery
Alcoholism and Other Drug
    Dependencies (AMSAODD)
Algology (Chronic Pain)
Alternative Medicine
Ambulatory Anesthesia
Ambulatory Foot Surgery
Anesthesia
Arthroscopic Surgery
Arthroscopy
    (Board of North America)

B

Bariatric Medicine
Bionic Psychology
Bloodless Medicine & Surgery

C

Chelation Therapy
Chemical Dependence
Clinical Chemistry
Clinical Ecology
Clinical Medicine and Surgery
Clinical Neurology
Clinical Neurosurgery
Clinical Nutrition
Clinical Orthopaedic Surgery
Clinical Pharmacology
Clinical Polysomnography
Clinical Psychiatry

Clinical Psychology
Clinical Toxicology
Cosmetic Plastic Surgery
Cosmetic Surgery
Council of Non-Board
    Certified Physicians
Critical Care in Medicine &
    Surgery

D

Dermalogy
Disability Analysis
Disability Evaluating Physicians

E

Electrodiagnostic Medicine
Electroencephalography
Electromyography &
    Electrodiagnosis
Environmental Medicine
Epidemiology (College)
Eye Surgery

F

Facial Cosmetic Surgery
Facial Plastic & Reconstructive
    Surgery
Forensic Examiners
Forensic Toxicology

H

Hand Surgery
Head, Facial & Neck Pain &
    TMJ Orthopaedics
Health Physics
Homeopathic Physicians

193

Plastic Esthetic Surgeons
Prison Medicine
Professional Disability
    Consultants Psychiatric
    Medicine
Psychiatry (American National
    Board of)
Psychoanalysis (American
    Examining Board in)
Psychological Medicine
    (International)

Q

Quality Assurance & Utilization
    Review

R

Radiology & Medical Imaging
Rheumatologic Surgery
Rheumatological &
    Reconstructive Medicine
Ringside Medicine & Surgery

S

Skin Specialists
Sleep Medicine
    (Polysomnography)
Spinal Cord Injury
Spinal Surgery
Sports Medicine/Surgery

T

Toxicology
Trauma Surgery
Traumatologic Medicine &
    Surgery
Tropical Medicine

U

Ultrasound Technology
Urologic Allied Health
    Professionals
Urological Surgery

W

Weight Reduction Medicine

Appendix C

RESOURCES - PROFESSIONAL ORGANIZATIONS

All of the information listed below was abstracted from the organization's literature or website.

DENTAL

American Academy of Cosmetic Dentistry (AACD)
5401 World Dairy Drive
Madison, WI 53718
(608) 222-8583 / Fax (608) 222-9540
(800) 543-9220
E-mail: info@aacd.com
www.aacd.com

While anyone can join the American Academy of Cosmetic Dentistry, becoming an accredited member is a rigorous process with experience and exams as important components. In order to be included on the AACD referral list, Fellow Accredited, Sustaining and General Members must have attended two of the four most recent annual conferences (a four-day scientific session). This four-year period is monitored beginning with each member's initial year of membership. To become an accredited member a cosmetic dentist must continue his/her education, take a written and oral exam and submit clinical cases and reports.

American Association of Oral and Maxillofacial Surgery (AAOMS)
9700 West Bryn Mawr Avenue
Rosemont, IL 60018-5701
(847) 678-6200
Email: inquiries@aaoms.org
www.aaoms.org

Members consist of oral and maxillofacial surgeons, who are dentists specializing in surgery of the mouth, face and jaw. After four years of dental school, OMS receive four to seven years of hospital-based surgical and medical training, preparing them to do a wide range of procedures including all types of surgery of both the bones and soft tissues of the face, mouth and neck. Many oral and maxillofacial surgeons earn a medical degree as well as a dental degree, and would be identified by MD, DDS. Members must be: certified as a Diplomat of the American

Board of Oral and Maxillofacial Surgery; a member of the American Dental Association; a graduate of advance oral and maxillofacial surgery education program accredited by the ADA; ethical, practicing in the United States of its possessions; a member of his/her OMS state society.

American Association of Orthodontists (AAO)
401 N. Lindbergh Blvd.
St. Louis, MO 63141-7816
(800) 424-2841 / Fax: (314) 997-1745.
Email: info@aaortho.org
www.aaortho.org

To become a member, a dentist must complete an accredited orthodontic program, be a member in good standing of the American Dental Association, and have a practice exclusively in orthodontics. The American Dental Association requires orthodontists to have at least two academic years of advanced specialty training in orthodontics in an accredited program, after graduation from dental school. There are 14,600 members.

American Dental Association (ADA)
211 E. Chicago Ave.
Chicago, IL 60611
(312) 440-2500 / Fax: (312) 440-7494
www.ada.org

The ADA today has more than 147,000 members 53 constituent (state-territorial) and 545 component (local) dental societies. Membership in the American Dental Association is available to all dentists and dental students in good standing. The association provides information to consumers about products and educational information to teachers and schools about dental care. It provides training seminars to dentists.

American Society of Maxillofacial Surgeons (ASMS)
ASMS Executive Office
4900B South 31st St.
Arlington, VA 22206-1656
(703) 820-7400 / Fax: (703) 931-4520
E-mail: admin@maxface.org
www.maxface.org

ASMS is the oldest American organization representing maxillofacial surgeons who are devoted to improving and promoting the highest levels of patient care. The members of the Society are surgeons who hold both the MD and DDS or DMD degrees, or only the MD degree. Members must: complete five years of recognized graduate training in preparation for maxillofacial surgery; be sponsored by an active or senior member, and endorsed by a second active or senior member; and be engaged in the practice of surgery in the same geographical area for a minimum of one year prior to proposal.

MEDICAL

American Academy of Cosmetic Surgery (AACS)
Cosmetic Surgery Information Service
737 N. Michigan Ave.
Suite 820
Chicago, IL 60611
(312) 981-6760
www.cosmeticsurgery.org

AACS is an accredited council of professionals devoted to post-graduate medical and educational opportunities in the field of cosmetic surgery. It is the nation's largest multidisciplinary medical association that exclusively devotes its educational efforts to cosmetic surgery. The membership is comprised of plastic surgeons, dermatologists and other specialists including maxillofacial surgeons and ophthalmologists. Membership may be granted to a physician (MD or DO) who is a resident of the United States of American or Canada, who has performed at least one hundred (100) cosmetic surgery procedures as the independent surgeon during a 1 year period prior to applying for admission as a Fellow, and is Board Certified in an ABMS approved surgical subspecialty including, but not limited to: Otolaryngology, Plastic and Reconstructive Surgery, Dermatology, Obstetrics/Gynecology, General Surgery, Cosmetic Surgery, Ophthalmology or Oral and Maxillofacial Surgery.

Subgroups of AACS:
>   American Society of Hair Restoration (ASHR)
>   American Society of Lipo-Suction Surgeons (ASLSS)

American Academy of Dermatology (AAD)
1350 I St. NW, Suite 880
Washington, DC 20005-4355
(202) 842-3555 / Fax: (202) 842-4355
www.aad.org

The American Academy of Dermatology is the largest, most influential and most representative of all dermatological associations. With a membership of more than

13,700, it represents virtually all practicing dermatologists in the United States. The academy has developed a platform to: promote and advance the science and art of medicine and surgery related to the skin; promote the highest possible standards in clinical practice, education and research in dermatology and related disciplines; and support and enhance patient care and promote the public interest relating to dermatology.

American Academy of Facial Plastic & Reconstructive Surgery (AAFPRS)
310 S. Henry Street
Alexandria, VA 22314
(703) 299-9291 / Fax (703) 299-8898
www.facial-plastic-surgery.org

To become a member physicians must be board certified in a specialty board recognized by the ABMS that focuses on the head and neck area or its equivalent. A majority of the members are certified by the American Board of Otolaryngology, which includes study in facial plastic surgery. Others are certified in plastic surgery, ophthalmology, and dermatology. A member must be: a diplomat of a recognized American examining board of medical specialties in a specialty applicable to the head, face and neck area, or its equivalent; a fellow in the American College of Surgeons or the Royal College of Surgeons; or a diplomat of the American Board of Facial Plastic and Reconstructive Surgery. Fellows must have training and experience in facial plastic and reconstructive surgery and have been in practice for three years. Members have to submit a detailed report of 35 major facial plastic and reconstructive surgical procedures performed within the past year.

American Academy of Otolaryngologists (AAO-HNS)
American Academy of Otolaryngolgy-HNS
One Prince St.
Alexandria, VA 22314
(703) 836-4444
www.ENTnet.org

The Academy represents more than 10,000 otolaryngologist--head and neck surgeons who diagnose and treat disorders of the ears, nose, throat, and related structures of the head and neck. The AAO-HNS Foundation works to advance the art, science and ethical practice of otolaryngology--head and neck surgery through education, research, and lifelong learning. Membership is open to any physician who holds a degree of Doctor of Medicine, Doctor of Osteopathy, or equivalent medical degree as determined by the Board of Directors of the Academy; who holds a valid and unrestricted license to practice medicine in the United States or

Canada. Only physicians who have been certified by a specialty board acceptable to the Board of Directors shall be eligible to become a Fellow.

American Association of Plastic Surgeons (AAPS)
www.aaps1921.org

To become a member of the AAPS, a physician must be certified by either the American Board of Plastic Surgery or the Royal College of Physicians and Surgeons of Canada in Plastic Surgery must certify members. Members are included by invitation only and candidates must show recognized contributions of quality in the field of plastic surgery as a pre-requisite to membership. They will be expected to have made outstanding contributions to the field of plastic surgery in the areas of education, research or clinical excellence.

American College of Surgeons (ACS)
633 N. Saint Clair St.
Chicago IL 60611-3211
(312) 202-5000 / Fax: (312) 202-5001
www.facs.org

The American College of Surgeons is a scientific and educational association of surgeons that was founded in 1913 to improve the quality of care for the surgical patient by setting high standards for surgical education and practice. Members of the American College of Surgeons are referred to as "Fellows." The letters FACS (Fellow, American College of Surgeons) after a surgeon's name mean that the surgeon's education and training, professional qualifications, surgical competence, and ethical conduct have passed a rigorous evaluation, and have been found to be consistent with the high standards established and demanded by the college.

American Medical Association (AMA)
515 North State Street
Chicago, IL 60610
(312) 464-5000
www.ama-assn.org

Founded more than 150 years ago, the AMA is the largest medical organization, which develops and promotes the standards in medical practice, research, and education; advocates on behalf of patients and physicians; and commits to provide timely information on matters important to the health of America. The AMA strives to serve as the voice of the American medical profession. The organization's policy is developed through a democratic process that brings together informed viewpoints on issues important to physicians and the patients they serve. The seat of

AMA policymaking is the AMA House of Delegates where state, local and specialty society representatives set policy through a consensus-building process. In addition, the AMA maintains information about physicians practicing throughout the nation. Healthcare consumers can use their database to check the location, licensing, education and specialty of many doctors in the United States. Physicians can use the website to learn about pending legislation, upcoming seminars, fellow physicians, medical breakthroughs, and discuss medical cases with one another.

American Society for Dermatologic Surgery (ASDS)
5550 Meadowbrook Dr.
Suite 120
Rolling Meadows, IL 60008
(847) 956-0900 / Fax: (847) 956-0999
Email: info@aboutskinsurgery.com
www.asds-net.org

The American Society for Dermatologic Surgery was founded in 1970 to promote excellence in the subspecialty of dermatologic surgery and foster the highest standards of patient care. With 3,500 members, ASDS is the largest subspecialty group in dermatology and represents the fastest growing segment of dermatologic practice. To become a member a physician must be certified by the American Board of Dermatology or in dermatology by the Royal College of Physicians and Surgeons in Canada.

American Society of Aesthetic Plastic Surgeons (ASAPS)
ASAPS Central Office
11081 Winners Circle
Los Alamitos, California 90720
(562) 799-2356 / Fax (562) 799-1098
(800)-364-2147
Email: asaps@surgery.org
www.surgery.org

ASAPS is an association of plastic surgeons, who must be certified in plastic surgery by the American Board of Plastic Surgeons. Only a fraction of ABPS plastic surgeons are members due to stringent requirements. There is a separate category of "Candidate" which is for less experienced ABMS certified plastic surgeons who may or may not be chosen to become members of ASAPS. There are 1,900 members in the U.S. and Canada. Membership is by invitation only.

American Society of Anesthesiologists (ASA)

520 N. Northwest Highway
Park Ridge, IL 60068-2573

(847) 825-5586 / Fax: (847) 825-1692
Email: mail@asahq.org
www.asahq.org

The American Society of Anesthesiologists is an educational, research and scientific association of physicians organized to raise and maintain the standards of the medical practice of anesthesiology and improve the care of the patient. Members of ASA must be Doctors of Medicine or Osteopathy who are licensed practitioners and have successfully completed a training program in anesthesiology approved by the Accreditation Council for Graduate Medical Education (ACGME) or the American Osteopathic Association (AOA). Members must maintain the high standards required by the Society throughout their careers.

American Society of Laser Medicine & Surgery (ASLMS)

2404 Stewart Avenue,
Wausau WI USA 54401

(715) 845-9283 / Fax: (715) 848-2493
Email: information@aslms.org
www.aslms.org

The American Society for Laser Medicine and Surgery is the world's largest scientific organization dedicated to promoting research, education and high standards of clinical care in the field of medical laser applications. The society has a broad base of membership including physicians and surgeons, nurses, and other health professionals involved in laser treatment of patients, physicists who develop devices, biomedical engineers who adapt them for medical purposes, and biologists who investigate the interaction of laser light with tissue. Any scientist, physician, other health care professional, or any individual who is qualified and duly licensed to engage in independent clinical practice and is qualified and recognized in his or her respective field, such as dentistry, dermatology, and other ABMS boards.

American Society of Ophthalmic Plastic & Reconstructive Surgery (ASOPRS)

Executive Office
1133 West Morse Blvd, #201
Winter Park, FL 32789
(407) 647-8839
www.asoprs.org.

The American Society of Ophthalmic Plastic and Reconstructive Surgery has more than 400 national and international members, who must complete an ASOPRS sponsored fellowship residency. The society was founded in 1969 to establish a qualified body of surgeons who have training and experience in this highly specialized field. The mission of this Society is to advance training, education, research, and the quality of clinical practice in the fields of aesthetic, plastic, and reconstructive surgery specializing in the face, eyelids, orbits, and lacrimal system.

American Society of Plastic Surgeons (ASPS)
Plastic Surgery Educational Foundation
444 E. Algonquin Rd.
Arlington Heights, IL 60005
Plastic Surgeon Referral Service
(888) 4-PLASTIC / (888) 475-2784)
www.plasticsurgery.org

ASPS comprise 97% of all physicians certified by the American Board of Plastic Surgery (ABSP). Plastic surgeons must be certified by the ABPS (in Canada by the Royal College of Physicians and Surgeons of Canada). All members have graduated from an accredited medical school, have had five years of residency (usually three years of general surgery followed by two years of plastic surgery residency), two year of post residency practice, and pass comprehensive and written exams. ASPS members are qualified to perform cosmetic and reconstructive surgical procedures – everything from liposuction to intricate reconstructive microsurgery.

The International Confederation of Plastic Reconstructive and Aesthetic Surgery (ICPRAS)
www.worldplasticsurgery.org

The IPRAS is a society comprised of more than 90 national plastic surgery societies from around the world, including the ASPS. The International Plastic, Reconstructive and Aesthetic Surgery Foundation is the Educational and Humanitarian Foundation of IPRAS. The society promotes worldwide learning including volunteering services in third-wold countries.

International Society of Hair Restoration Surgery (ISHRS)
13 South 2nd Street
Geneva, IL 60134 USA
(630) 262-5399 / Fax: (630) 262-1520
(800) 444-2737
Email: info@ishrs.org
www.ishrs.org

The International Society of Hair Restoration Surgery (ISHRS) is a non-profit voluntary organization of over 700 hair restoration specialists around the world. It was founded in 1992 as the first International society to promote Continuing Quality Improvement and education for professionals in the field of hair restoration surgery. Members should be of good moral character and be in good standing in their community, and are fully licensed to practice medicine with an interest in hair restoration and scalp surgery.

Society of Plastic Surgical Skin Care Specialists
SPSSCS Central Office
11081 Winners Circle, Suite 200
Los Alamitos, CA 90720-2813
(562) 799-0466 / Fax: (562) 799-1098
(800) 486-0611
www.surgery.org/skincare

In 1994, a group of renowned plastic surgeons recognized the need to provide an educational forum for the emerging specialty of plastic surgical skin care. The SPSSCS was created from this vision and now serves as the professional organization to promote and educate plastic surgical skin care professionals worldwide.

The SPSSCS offers membership opportunities for licensed plastic surgical skin care specialists practicing in the offices of Board Certified Plastic Surgeons. Membership is open to registered nurses, licensed practical nurses or licensed skin care professionals practicing under the direct supervision of a plastic surgeon certified by or eligible for examination by the ABPS or the Royal College of Physicians and Surgeons of Canada.

OTHER HEALTHCARE

The Accreditation Association for Ambulatory Health Care (AAAHC)
3201 Old Glenview Road, Suite 300
Wilmette, Illinois 60091-2992
(847) 853-6060 / Fax: (847) 853-9028
www.aaahc.org.

The AAAHC is a leader in ambulatory health care accreditation and serves as an advocate for the provision and documentation of high quality health services in ambulatory health care organizations. This is accomplished through the development of standards and through its survey and accreditation programs.

The American Association for Accreditation of Ambulatory Surgery (AAAAS)
1202 Allanson Road
Mundelein, IL 60060
(888) 545-5222 / Fax: (847) 566-4580
www.AAAASF.org.

The American Association for Accreditation of Ambulatory Surgery Facilities (AAAASF) is a voluntary program of inspection and accreditation in surgery facilities to ensure excellence and quality care to patients.

American Association of Nurse Anesthetists (AANA)
222 S. Prospect Avenue
Park Ridge, IL 60068-4001
(847) 692-7050 / Fax: 847-692-6968
www.aana.com

Anesthesia is a recognized specialty in nursing. Founded in 1931, AANA is the professional association representing more than 28,000 Certified Registered Nurse Anesthetists (CRNAs) nationwide. The AANA promulgates education, and practice standards and guidelines, and affords consultation to both private and governmental entities regarding nurse anesthetists and their practice.

American Board of Medical Specialties (ABMS)
1007 Church Street, Suite 404
Evanston, Illinois 60201-5913
(847) 491-9091 / Fax (847) 328-3596
(866) ASK-ABMS
www.abms.org

The ABMS is the authoritative body for the recognition of medical specialties, coordinating 24 medical specialty boards (including 25 medical specialties) and providing information on the board certification of doctors.

American Hospital Association (AHA)
1 North Franklin
Chicago, IL 60606
(312) 422-2000 / (800) 424-4301
www.aha.org

A national health advocacy organization, the AHA represents hospitals and healthcare networks in legislative and regulatory matters. In 1973 the AHA adopted the Patient Bill of Rights to help patients understand their rights and responsibilities.

American Osteopathic Association (AOA)
142 E. Ontario St.
Chicago, IL 60611
(800) 621-1773
www.aoa-net.org

The AOA is the national organization for the advancement of osteopathic medicine in the United States, and the professional association for more than 48,000 physicians. The AOA accredits the Colleges of Osteopathic Medicine, osteopathic internship and residency programs, and healthcare facilities.

Joint Commission on Accreditation of Healthcare Organizations (JCAHO)
(630) 792-5800
www.jcaho.org

The Joint Commission (JCAHO) is an independent, not-for-profit organization, which evaluates the quality and safety of care for nearly 17,000 health care organizations. To maintain and earn accreditation, organizations must have an extensive on-site review by a team of JCAHO health care professionals, at least once every three years. JCAHO is governed by a board that includes physicians, nurses, and consumers. JCAHO sets the standards by which health care quality is measured in America and around the world.

Appendix D

The Internet is an ideal place to find a doctor or check on your doctor's credentials, but you have to know where to look and what pitfalls to avoid. There is a plethora of websites that claim to be official and offer advice; some are commercial, while others are run by hospitals, governments, health plans or physician organizations. However, there are pervasive problems with the quality, quantity, and accuracy of information on physician directory websites. Some individual sites include only a minimal amount of information, such as medical school and specialty board certification. The prevailing snag with many websites is a lack of up-to-date and detailed information, and evidence that the data has been verified. Considering the power of the Internet to search data, we have compiled a list of the key websites that offer sound information and profile qualified cosmetic doctors and dentists. These sites are essential tools in educating and empowering consumers to make informed decisions.

Dentistry & Oral Surgery

www.aacd.com – American Academy of Cosmetic Dentistry

www.estheticacademy.org – American Academy of Esthetic Dentistry

www.aaoms.org – American Association of Oral and Maxillofacial Surgeons

www.aaortho.org – American Association of Orthodontists

www.ada.org – American Dental Association

www.orthodontics.com – American Orthodontic Society

Cosmetic Surgery & Dermatology

www.cosmeticsurgery.org – American Academy of Cosmetic Surgery

www.aad.org – American Academy of Dermatology

www.ENTnet.org – American Academy of Otolaryngologists

www.aafprs.org – American Academy of Facial and Reconstructive Plastic Surgeons

www.aaoms.org – American Association of Oral and Maxillofacial Surgeons

www.abderm.org – American Board of Dermatology

www.aboto.org – American Board of Otolarygology

www.abplsurg.org – American Board of Plastic Surgery

www.asds-net.org – American Society for Dermatologic Surgery

www.asoprs.org – American Society of Ophthalmic Plastic and Reconstructive Surgeons

www.surgery.org – American Society for Aesthetic Plastic Surgery

www.plasticsurgery.org – American Society of Plastic Surgeons

www.plasticsurgery.ca – The Canadian Society of Plastic Surgeons

www.worldplasticsurgery.org – International Confederation for Plastic Reconstructive and Aesthetic Surgery

www.inhrs.org – International Society of Hair Restoration Surgery

General

www.aaaasf.org – American Association for Accreditation of Ambulatory Surgery Facilities

www.aaahc.org – Accreditation Association for Ambulatory Health Care

www.abms.org – American Board of Medical Specialties

www.facs.org – American College of Surgeons

www.ama-assn.org – American Medical Association

www.aoa-net.org – American Osteopathic Association

www.asahq.org – American Society of Anesthesiologists

www.aslms.org – American Society for Laser Medicine & Surgery

www.fsmb.org – Federation of State Medical Boards

www.jcaho.org – Joint Commission on Accreditation of Healthcare Organizations

Appendix E

CHECKLISTS

1 YOUR MEDICAL HISTORY

N.B. *(Complete and bring along with you to consultations so you don't leave anything out)*

NAME _____

Date of Birth _____ Age _____

Height _____

Weight _____

LIST ALL PREVIOUS SURGERY WITH DATES:

Operation   Surgeon   Date

_____

_____

_____

_____

_____

_____

_____

_____

_____

Do you have a history of:

☐ Asthma

☐ Bleeding Disorders

☐ Cancer

☐ Keloid or hypertrophic scars

☐ Excessive bruising

☐ Bronchitis, Chronic cough

☐ Tuberculosis

☐ Radio Therapy

☐ Hernia

☐ Shortness of breath

☐ Hypertension

☐ Blood clots

☐ Headaches

☐ Cold sores, Herpes

☐ Hepatitis A B C

☐ Mitral Valve Prolapse,
   Heart Murmur

☐ Drug Abuse

☐ Alcoholism

☐ Nose Bleeds

☐ Thyroid Disease

☐ Dry Eye

☐ Seizures

☐ Depression

☐ Facial Paralysis

☐ Osteo or Rheumatoid Arthritis

☐ Lupus or Auto Immune Disease

In the past year, have you taken:

☐ Blood pressure medication

☐ Cardiac medication

☐ Diet pills

☐ Diuretics

☐ Vitamins, Herbal supplements

☐ Tranquilizers

☐ Alcohol

☐ Sleeping pills

☐ Anti-depressants

☐ Pain medication

☐ Accutane®

☐ Estrogen Replacement Therapy

☐ Aspirin or other anti-inflammatories

Have you had an adverse reaction to:

☐ Anesthesia

☐ Diabetes

☐ Antibiotics

☐ Codeine

☐ Demerol

☐ Adhesive tape

☐ Aspirin

☐ Sulphur

☐ Penicillin

☐ Valium

☐ Iodine

☐ Morphine

☐ Suture material

211

LIST ANY ALLERGIES TO MEDICATIONS:

_____

_____

_____

_____

_____

LIST ALL MEDICATIONS INCLUDING OTC THAT YOU ARE TAKING WITH DOSAGES:

Drug	Dosage	No. Times Per Day

Name of Internist: _____

Hospital Affiliation: _____

Address: _____

Telephone: _____

Fax: _____

Name of Any Specialists: _____

Specialty: _____

Address: _____

Telephone: _____

Fax: _____

2 CONSULTATION NOTES

DOCTOR

Tel

Office Address

Secretary/Nurse

DIAGNOSIS (the doctor's findings)

TREATMENT PLAN (check all that apply)

☐ Botulinum Toxin

☐ Fat transfer

☐ Liposuction of the neck

☐ Lower lid fat removal

☐ Upper lid skin, fat removal

☐ Endoscopic brow lift

☐ Open forehead lift

☐ Temporal or upper face-lift

☐ Mid face-lift or cheek lift

☐ Lip augmentation

☐ Chin implant

☐ Lower facelift

☐ Endoscopic face-lift

☐ Face and necklift

☐ Composite face-lift

☐ Subperiosteal lift

☐ Resurfacing – Erbium:YAG

☐ Resurfacing – Carbon Dioxide

☐ OTHER

PROCEDURE PERFORMED *(circle)*

Hospital   Office   Operating Room   Surgicenter

NAME OF HOSPITAL:

ANESTHESIA *(circle)*   Local   Twilight   General

FEES:

Surgeon   _____

Anesthesiologist   _____

Hospital   _____

Implants   _____

OTHER   _____

TOTAL:

Photos: (circle)   taken   to be arranged

LEAD TIME FOR SURGERY DATE: (CIRCLE)

up to 4 weeks   4-8 weeks   8-12 weeks   3-6 months   6 months+

Deposit amount:

Deposit due:

Balance due:

NOTES:

_____

_____

_____

_____

3 PRE SURGERY CHECKLIST

1 month before

☐ Go for your preoperative blood tests, EKG, Chest X-ray

☐ For facial surgery, have your last hair trim before surgery keeping hair long around the ears

☐ Start an active anti-aging vitamin A,E,C-enriched skincare regimen

☐ OTHER

3 weeks before

☐ Stop all aspirin and other drugs that cause bleeding

☐ Avoid multi-vitamins, Vitamin E and natural supplements that may cause bleeding

☐ Go off cigarettes and nicotine substitutes entirely

☐ OTHER

2 weeks before

☐ If requested, discontinue hormone replacement therapy

☐ Load up on Vitamin C (1,000 - 1,500mg/day)

☐ Cut down on alcohol

☐ OTHER

1 week before

☐ Last chance for highlights or coloring your hair

☐ Pick up a camouflage cream and green undertone for concealing bruises

☐ Get supplies from pharmacy (gloves, gauzes, hydrogen peroxide, swabs, etc.)

☐ Have any prescriptions filled

☐ Get your brows waxed or plucked

☐ Arrange to have a friend or family member take you home after surgery

☐ OTHER

The day before

- ☐ Stock up on broth, juices, water, teas, soft foods
- ☐ Pack your hospital bag if needed with night gown or pajamas, slippers, toothbrush
- ☐ Start your Arnica tablets or capsules, if your doctor prescribed it
- ☐ Begin your antibiotics, if instructed to do so
- ☐ Buy a good book, your favorite magazines, rent a few videos
- ☐ Call your surgeon's office to confirm the time to arrive at hospital
- ☐ Schedule your first postop visit
- ☐ OTHER

The night before

- ☐ Remove nail polish only if requested, and contact lenses
- ☐ Set your alarm
- ☐ Enjoy a leisurely dinner avoiding highly salted or spiced foods
- ☐ Wash your hair twice
- ☐ Nothing to eat or drink after midnight
- ☐ Fill all of the ice trays in the freezer
- ☐ OTHER

The morning of

- ☐ Wear loose-fitting clothes and nothing that pulls over your head
- ☐ Wash your face and brush your teeth
- ☐ Don't apply moisturizer, body lotion, fragrance or makeup
- ☐ Change the bed linens to old ones and fluff your pillows
- ☐ Arrange your bedside tray with everything you will need
- ☐ Leave your jewels and wristwatch at home
- ☐ OTHER

YOUR MEDICATION CHART

7 DAY MEDICATION CHART

Label all your medications so you don't get confused, and keep them together at your bedside on a tray.

Enter day to start and finish, i.e. Day 1, 2, etc., and check off what times of day to take.

	START	AM	MID DAY	PM	BEDTIME	FINISH
Antibiotic Name:						
Pain pills Name:						
Anti viral Name:						
Sleep aid Name:						
Vitamin/ Supplement Name:						
Eye Lubricant/ Drops Name:						
OTHER(S):						

5 MEDICATIONS TO DISCONTINUE

GUIDELINES FOR MEDICATIONS TO BE DISCONTINUED PRIOR TO SURGERY *This is only a partial list. Consult with your doctor before discontinuing any medication.*

ASPIRIN COMBINATIONS

- Ascriptin
- Aspergum
- Bufferin
- Darvon
- Easprin
- Ecotrin
- Exedrin
- Fiornal
- Lortab
- Norgesic

ASPIRIN WITH ANTACID

- Alka-Seltzer

ANTI-INFLAMMATORIES

- Advil
- Aleve
- Anacin
- Anaprox
- Bayer
- Bufferin
- Cataflam
- Clinoril
- Dolobid
- Empirin
- Entab-650
- Feldene
- Ibuprofen
- Indocin
- Indomethacin
- Lodine
- Midol
- Nalfon
- Ponstel
- Relafen

ANTI-PYRETICS

- Aleve
- Feverall
- Trilisate

ARTHRITIS MEDICATIONS

- Aleve
- Anaprox
- Ansaid
- Blocadren
- Cafergot
- Cataflam
- Clinoril
- Darvon
- Daypro
- Solganal
- Dolobid
- Ecotrin
- Ergomar
- Ergostat
- Feldene
- Fiorinal
- Imitrex
- Indocin
- Lodine
- Midrin
- Migrilam
- Mono-gesic
- Motrin
- Myochrysine
- Naprosyn
- Orudis
- Oruvail
- Ridaura
- Sal-flex
- Telectin
- Toradol
- Voltaren
- Wigraine

PLATELET INHIBITORS

- Aspirin
- Baby Aspirin
- Bufferin
- Halfprin
- Persantine
- Ticlid

TOPICAL PREPARATIONS

- Absorbent
- Absorbine
- Act-on-Rub
- Ben Gay
- Doan's Rub
- Exocaine Plus
- HEET
- Icy Hot
- Infrarub
- Metholatum
- Neurabain
- Oil-O-Sol
- Panagesic
- Sloan's
- Solitice
- Stimurub
- Surin
- Yager's Lin.
- Zemo Liquid

COLD MEDICATIONS 4-WAY COLD

- Alka-Seltzer
- Dristan
- Quiet World
  Analgesic
- Sine-off
- St. Joseph's
  for Children
- Vanquish

VITAMINS AND SUPPLEMENTS

- Echinacea
- Ephedra
- Garlic
- Gingko
  Biloba
- Ginseng
- Mah Huang
- St Johns Wort
- Vitamin E

OTHER PRODUCTS CONTAINING ASPIRIN

- ACA Caps
- APAC Acetonyl
- Aidant
- Alka Seltezer
- Allygesic
- Apamead
- APC
- Aphodyne
- Aphophen
- Arthra-Zene
- ASA
- Asalco
- Ascaphen
- As-ca-phen
- ACD Acetabar
- Acetasem
- Aprine
- Aluprin
- Amosodyne
- Amytal
- Anacin
- Amytal
- Anexsia
- Anadynos
- Ascodeen
- Ascriptin
- Aspadine
- Aspergum
- Aspac
- Aspencaf
- Aspyte
- Aspirbar
- Aspir-C
- Aspireze
- Aspirin (USP)
- Aluminum
- Children's Aspirin
- Aspircal
- Aspir-phen
- Axotal
- Babylove
- Bayer
- Bayer Timed-Release
- Brogesic
- Bufabar
- Buff-A
- Buffacetin
- Buff-a-comp
- Buffadyne
- Bufferin
- Buffinol
- Calurin
- Cama Inlay
- Capron
- Causalin
- Cephalgesic
- Cheracol
- Cirin
- Clistanal
- Codasa
- Codempiral
- Codesal
- Coldate
- Colrex
- Congesprin
- Cope
- Coralson
- Modified Cordex
- Coricidin
- Co-ryd
- Counter pain
- Covangesic
- Darvon
- Darvon with ASA
- Darvon Compound
- Davo-Tran
- Dasikon
- Dasin Caps
- Decagesic
- Delenar
- Derfort
- Derfule
- Dolcin
- Dolene
- Dolor
- Doloral
- Dorodal
- Drinacet
- Dristan
- Drocogesic
- Duopac
- Duradyne
- Ecotrin
- Empiral
- Empirin

OTHER PRODUCTS CONTAINING ASPIRIN CONTINUED

- Emprazil
- Duragesic
- Empragen
- Equagesic
- Excedrin
- Fiorinal
- Fizrin
- Formasal
- Fizrin
- Formasal 4 way Cold Tabs
- Gelsodyne
- Grillodyne
- Hasamal CT
- Henasphen
- Histadyl
- Hypan
- I-Pac
- Kryl
- Liquiprin
- Lumasprin
- Marnal
- Measurin
- Medadent
- Medaprin
- Midol
- Midol 200
- Multihist
- Nembudeine
- Nembu-Gesic
- Nipirin
- Norgesic

- Novahistine
- Novrad
- Opacedrin
- Opasal
- Paadon
- Pabirin
- PAC
- Palgesic
- PC-65
- Pedidyne
- Pentagesic
- Pentagill
- Percobarb
- Percodan
- Persistin
- Phac Tab
- Phenaphen
- Phencaset
- Phenergan
- Phenodyne
- Pheno-Formasal
- Phensal
- Pirseal
- Palygesic
- Ponodyne
- Predisal
- Prolaire-B
- Pyrasal
- Pyrhist Cold
- Pyrroxate
- Phinex
- Robaxisal

- Ryd
- Sal-Aceto
- Sal-Fayne
- Salibar Jr
- Salipral
- Sarogesic
- Sedalgesic
- Semaldyne
- Sigmagen
- Sine-Off
- Spirin Buffered
- Stanback
- Ster-Darvon
- St. Joseph
- Supac
- Super-Anahist
- Synalgos
- Synirin
- Tetrex-APC
- Thephorin-AC
- Toloxidyne
- Trancogesic
- Trancoprin
- Triaminicin
- Trigesic
- Triocin
- Vanquish
- Zactirim
- Zorpin
- Feldene
- Indocin

Appendix F

The following is a list of terms from the text of the book and others you may come across when discussing procedures with your doctor or dentist.

A

Abdominoplasty Plastic surgery of the abdomen in which excess fatty tissue and skin are removed.

Ablation Vaporization of the most superficial layers of skin.

Abutment A tooth or root that is used to anchor a bridge.

Acne A chronic skin condition characterized by an inflammatory eruption of the skin that occurs when a hair follicle gets plugged with sebum and dead cells. Rising hormone levels stimulate oil glands, which cause clogged pores and inflammation.

Actinic Keratosis (Solar keratosis) a lesion that is dry, scaly, rough, and tan or pink caused by sun exposure, considered precancerous.

Alar Base The wing-like structures at the base of the nose

Allergen A substance that can cause allergic reaction.

Allograft A graft from the same species as the recipient, as in human skin.

Alopecia A condition of hair loss.

Alpha Hydroxy Acid (AHA) A group of acids derived from foods such as fruit and milk, which can improve the texture of the skin by removing layers of dead cells and encouraging cell regeneration. There are many AHA's but the most common forms are Lactic Acid, Glycolic Acid, Pyruvic Acid, Tartaric Acid and Maleic Acid.

Amalgam Silver colored metal tooth filling material made from zinc, silver, tin, copper and mercury.

Anatomic Breast Implant Teardrop-shaped implant as opposed to the round style designed to look more like a natural breast.

Anemia A pathological deficiency in the oxygen-carrying component of the blood, measured in unit volume concentrations of hemoglobin, red blood cell volume, or red blood cell number.

Anti-oxidant A substance designed to prevent a chemical reaction with oxygen, e.g. Vitamins C, E, A, grape seed, green tea.

Areola The pigmented skin around the nipple.

Arnica A botanical derived from a mountain plant with antiseptic, astringent, antimicrobial and anti-inflammatory properties.

Autologous Occurring naturally in a certain type of tissue of the body.

B

Banana Roll The 'roll' of fat directly situated beneath the buttock crease.

Beta HCG Human Chorionic Gonadotropin. The "pregnancy hormone" is produced by the placenta.

Beta Hydroxy Acid (Salicylic Acid) A family of acids that enhance cell renewal, found naturally in willow bark.

Bleaching Agents Substances which slow down or block the production of melanin to lighten age spots and fade areas of hyperpigmentation; i.e. Hydroquinone, Kojic Acid, Azelaic Acid.

Blepharitis Inflammation of the eyelids characterized by redness and swelling and dried crusts.

Blepharoplasty (Eyelid Plasty) Surgery that removes excess fat, muscle, and/or skin around the eyes. Incisions follow the natural contour lines of the upper and lower lids, or can be done through the lining of the lower eyelid, providing access to skin and fatty issue.

Bonding Adhering a tooth colored substance to repair and/or change the color or shape of a tooth.

Botulinium Toxin A naturally occurring toxin that is injected into facial muscles to temporarily paralyze them and eliminate expression lines of the face, around the eyes, and the neck.

Bridge Dental appliance that can be fixed or moveable; used to replace missing or lost teeth.

Buffer An additive that adjusts the pH balance of a skin preparation

Buccal fat pads Fat pads located in the cheek.

C

CAD/CAM Acronym for computer assisted design/computer assisted manufacture technology. Data is supplied through imaging or by tracing the tooth, which allows the dentist to make veneers, onlays and inlays.

Cannulae Long, thin hollow tubular instrument used to extract fat during liposuction.

Capillary The smallest type of blood vessel in the body. Spider veins, for instance, are actually small capillaries commonly found on the face or legs.

Capsular Contracture Scar tissue that forms in the pocket surrounding a breast implant and becomes hardened and distorted.

Carbon Dioxide Laser technology that can be used to resurface moderate to deep facial wrinkles, scars, and can also be used as a cutting tool.

CAT Scan An image produced by a CAT scanner. Also called CT scan.

Catheter A hollow flexible tube for insertion into a body cavity, duct, or vessel to allow the passage of fluids or distend a passageway. Its uses include the drainage of urine from the bladder through the urethra or insertion through a blood vessel into the heart for diagnostic purposes.

Cauterize To burn or sear abnormal tissue with a cautery or caustic instrument, such as a laser.

CBC Complete Blood Count. The determination of the quantity of each type of blood cell in a given sample of blood, often including the amount of hemoglobin, the hematocrit, and the proportions of various white cells.

Cellulite Deposits of fat, toxins and fluids trapped in pockets beneath the skin, more common in women.

Cheek lift See mid-face-lift.

Chemical Peel A procedure in which a solution of varying strengths is applied to the entire face or to specific areas, such as around the mouth, to peel away the skin's top layers. Common peeling agents are Alpha Hydroxy Acid, Beta Hydroxy Acid, Trichloracetic Acid (TCA), Jessner's Solution, and Phenol.

Co Enzyme Q10 A renewal agent that stimulates natural cell energy production and regenerates Vitamin E.

Collagen A primary component of human skin that gives it resiliency, suppleness and tone, and breaks down with age due to muscle movement and environmental damage.

Columella The strip of skin dividing the nostrils at the base of the nose.

Comedones Open (blackheads) and closed (whiteheads) formed when pores become clogged with natural oils and impurities.

Commissure The area where two anatomic parts meet, as in the corner of the eye or the lips, typically referring to a fold or crease.

Composite Resin Plastic filling materials to which a filler has been added to increase strength.

Computer Imaging The use of a computer enhanced image to allow a doctor or dentist to illustrate how you may look after treatment, used as a patient education tool.

Congenital Defect Abnormality formed at birth.

Cornea The transparent convex anterior portion of the outer fibrous coat of the eyeball that covers the iris and the pupil and is continuous with the sclera.

Corneal Abrasion A scratch of the cornea of the eye.

Coronal Of or pertaining to the top of the head or skull.

Corrugator Muscle that is responsible for causing the glabellar or vertical lines that form between the eyebrows.

Cosmeceutical A substance that falls between the classification of a drug and a cosmetic, i.e., non-prescription over-the-counter formulations that provide pharmaceutical benefits.

Craniofacial surgery Surgery of the face and head.

Crust Surface layer formed by the drying of a bodily secretion.

Cuspid The canines, or teeth located in the corner of the arch, or third tooth on either side of the midline.

D

Deflation A rupture or tear in the shell of a breast implant that causes the filler (saline, silicone gel, or other) to leak out and the implant to flatten.

Dental Implants A manufactured material placed in or on the jawbone to aid in replacing missing teeth.

Dentin The main, calcareous part of a tooth, beneath the enamel and surrounding the pulp chamber and root canals.

Dermabrasion Non-surgical resurfacing procedure in which a hand-held rotary wheel is used to remove the top layer of skin.

Dermal fillers A category of substances that are either injected or implanted to shape and form overlying tissue.

Dermatitis An inflammatory condition of the skin that is characterized by itching and redness. Three categories of dermatitis are atopic, contact and seborrheic.

Dermis The layer of skin composed of collagen and elastin, lying beneath the epidermis (outer layer) and above the subcutaneous layers.

Diastema A space between two teeth.

Diode Contact laser technology that cuts and coagulates tissue.

Dry Eye A condition of the eyelids which causes dryness, blurred vision and the eyes to feel gritty.

Dystonia Abnormal tonicity of muscle, characterized by prolonged, repetitive muscle contractions that may cause twisting or jerking movements of the body or a body part.

E

Ecchymosis The passage of blood from ruptured blood vessels into subcutaneous tissue, marked by a purple discoloration of the skin.

Echinacea A natural substance thought to boost the immune system, and have anti-itching and soothing properties.

Ectropion A condition of the lower eyelid in which the lid is pulled downward from loose eyelid skin, muscles or too much skin having been removed, also called 'lid retraction'.

Eczema A chronic skin condition that superficial inflation in areas of the skin and scalp.

EKG Electrocardiograph. An instrument used in the detection and diagnosis of heart abnormalities that measures electrical potentials on the body surface and generates a record of the electrical currents associated with heart muscle activity.

Elastin A protein that is similar to collagen and the chief constituent of elastic fibers, also used as a surface protective agent in cosmetics to alleviate dry skin.

Electrolysis Use of electric current to permanently destroy the hair's root bulb.

Electrocautery To burn tissue with an electric current by use of a specially designed apparatus.

Electromyograph An instrument used in the diagnosis of neuromuscular disorders that produces an audio or visual record of the electrical activity of a skeletal muscle by means of an electrode inserted into the muscle or placed on the skin.

Electromyography The diagnosis of neuromuscular disorders with the use of an electromyograph.

Enamel The intensely hard calcified tissue entering into the composition of teeth.

Encapsulation The act of inclosing in a capsule; the growth of a membrane around (any part) so as to inclose it in a capsule.

Endoscopic Pertaining to an endoscope, an instrument for visualizing the interior of a hollow organ.

Endoscopic Surgery An endoscope is an small rigid tube-like instrument equipped with fiberoptic lighting, which can be introduced into the body through a tiny incision so that it lights up the surgical area. The surgeon can see the area on a video monitor while performing an operation, as in endoscopic browlifting, breast augmentation, face-lifting and tummy tucks.

Endosseous Another name for root-form implant. A dental implant, which is placed in the bone.

Endosteal Another name for root-form implant. A dental implant, which is placed in the bone.

Epidermis The outermost layer of the skin.

Epidural blocks Regional anesthesia resulting from injection of an anesthetic into the epidural space of the spinal cord; sensation is lost in the abdominal and genital and pelvic areas; used in childbirth and gynecological surgery.

Epinephrine A white to brownish crystalline compound isolated from the adrenal glands of certain mammals or synthesized and used in medicine as a heart stimulant, vasoconstrictor, and bronchial relaxant.

Epithelialization Regeneration of the epithelium or superficial layer of the skin, as occurs after laser resurfacing

Erbium: YAG A type of ablative laser that produces energy in a wavelength that penetrates the skin, is readily absorbed by water (a major component of tissue cells), and scatters the heat effects of the laser light.

Erythema Redness of the skin, as in post laser or other resurfacing, etc.

Exfoliant A material that removes dead surface skin cells.

Exfoliation To remove a layer of skin in flakes; peel.

External Ultrasound Utilizing ultrasonic energy applied externally to the skin to dissolve or liquefy fat deposits prior to liposuction.

Extrusion The erosion of skin that causes an implant (chin, lip, breast, etc.) to become partially exposed.

F

Face-lift See rhytidectomy

Fascia The sheet of connective tissue that covers the muscles, sometimes used as a graft material.

Fat Embolus Globules of fat that can infiltrate the bloodstream during surgery causing a mass that can result in serious complication and death.

Fibrin sealant A natural agent for the achievement of rapid hemostasis and tissue sealing in a variety of surgical applications. Also referred to as Tissue Glue.

Fibroblast A cell from which connective tissue develops.

Filler A category of substances that are either injected or implanted to shape and form overlying tissue. Common fillers are Bovine collagen, the patient's own fat or collagen from skin, human donor collagen.

Follicle A sheath that surrounds the root of the hair.

Forehead Lift Also called a browlift, pulls up droopy brows and upper lids, and improves wrinkling and vertical and horizontal frown lines. The Open Forehead Lift is more invasive than the Endoscopic Browlift. An 'Open' means that you will have an incision placed at or behind the ear through which excess skin is removed and muscles are tightened. An 'Endoscopic' lift is from 3 - 5 tiny incisions (1/2 - 1 inch) placed behind the hairline to remove muscles that cause frowning and wrinkles and/or elevate your brows.

Free Radicals A destructive form of oxygen generated by each cell in the body that destroys cellular membranes.

Frontalis The muscle that enables the brows to move up and down, and contributes to the formation of horizontal wrinkles of the forehead.

G

Gangrene Death and decay of body tissue, often occurring in a limb, caused by insufficient blood supply and usually following injury or disease.

General Anesthesia Commonly referred to as 'being asleep', a total loss of consciousness is induced by an anesthetist or anesthesiologist. The patient doesn't feel anything, and a breathing tube is placed in the airway.

Genioplasty To add projection to the chin, the bones are broken so that the chin area can be moved forward and secured in place.

Glabella The area between the eyebrows in the center of the forehead where deep vertical lines and creases often develop.

Graft A piece of tissue that is totally removed from one part of the body and transferred to another area of the body, as in fat, cartilage, bone, skin, etc.

Glaucoma Any of a group of eye diseases characterized by abnormally high intraocular fluid pressure, damaged optic disk, hardening of the eyeball, and partial to complete loss of vision.

Glycerin Used in moisturizers due to its water binding capabilities.

Glycolic acid an organic substace, found naturally in unripe grapes and in the leaves of the wild grape, and produced artificially in many ways, as by the oxidation of glycol.

Graves' Disease A condition usually caused by excessive production of thyroid hormone and characterized by an enlarged thyroid gland, protrusion of the eyeballs, a rapid heartbeat, and nervous excitability.

Gynecomastia Male breast reduction procedure usually accomplished via liposuction through small incisions in the areola and/or chest wall.

H

Hemangioma A benign skin lesion consisting of dense, usually elevated masses of dilated blood vessels.

Hematologist A doctor who specializes in diseases of the blood and blood-forming organs.

Hematoma A localized accumulation of blood in the skin caused by a blood vessel wall rupture, possible complication of surgery that may have to be drained.

Homeopathy A method of treating disease with naturally occurring substances.

Hyaluronic Acid An acid found naturally in the body and helps retain the skin's natural moisture.

Hydroquinone A bleaching agent that slows down or blocks the production of melanin to lighten age spots and to fade darkness and blotchiness.

Hydrochloric acid an aqueous solution of hydrogen chloride; a strongly corrosive acid.

Hyperpigmentation Darkening of certain skin areas through overproduction of melanin.

Hypertrophic Scar Thickened, raised or red scar tissue.

Hypertrophy Enlarged or thickened area.

Hypoallergenic A substance with a low chance of causing allergy or skin irritation.

Hypopigmentation Reduction in the pigment cells in the skin resulting in skin lightening.

Hypoplasia Incomplete or arrested development of an organ or a part.

Hypothyroidsim A glandular disorder resulting from insufficient production of thyroid hormones.

I

Incisor Central or lateral teeth with cutting edges, or the four front teeth, two on the upper and two on the lower.

Inframammary Crease The skin crease or fold that lies beneath the breast.

Inframammary Below the mammary gland.

Inlay Porcelain filling that is made to fit into a cavity and cemented into place, formely made from metals.

Isolagen An autologous filler fashioned from collagen from your own skin that is grown in a laboratory, processed and liquefied for later injection into wrinkles and folds.

J

Jaw Used to describe the maxillae and mandible and soft tissue surrounding the bony structure.

Jessner's Solution Pronounced 'yes-nerz', a pre-measured solution formulated with Resorcinol, Salicylic Acid, Lactic Acid with Ethanol originally developed by Dr. Max Jessner at New York University Hospital for the treatment of acne.

K

Keloid Enlarged, permanent and thickened scar formations that are more common in darker skin types, and often run in families.

Keratin A surface protective agent with film-forming and moisturizing action.

Kojic Acid Natural skin-lightening agent derived from a Japanese mushroom.

L

Lactic Acid A component of the skin's natural moisturizing factor.

Lagopthalmus Upper eyelid retraction that results in the difficulty of closing the upper eyelids.

Laminates The placement of a thin covering over discolored or broken teeth to improve their appearance.

L-ascorbic Acid The purest form of Vitamin C, which when applied topically is an anti-oxidant, anti-irritant, anti-inflammatory. It helps prevent wrinkles and age spots, stimulates collagen and brightens the skin.

Lateral Hooding Excess fold of skin between the eyebrow and the outer portion of the upper eyelid.

Lentigo Benign tan or brown colored lesion on the skin from sun exposure

Lidocaine A local anesthetic (trade name Xylocaine) used topically on the skin and mucous membranes.

Local Anesthesia Medications (usually in the 'caine' family) that are injected into a surgical or treatment site to cause temporary localized numbness.

Lymphatic System A network of structures, including ducts and nodes that carry lymph fluid from tissues to the bloodstream.

M

Malar Bags The pouch of loose skin and fluid that sometimes occurs with age below the lower eyelid area.

Malar Fat Pad A structure that sits in the second layer of the face below the cheekbone that is frequently positioned during facial rejuvenation procedures.

Malarplasty Cheekbone reduction or augmentation.

Malic Acid A glycolic acid derived from apples.

Malocclusion Faulty contact between the upper and lower teeth when the jaw is closed.

Mammogram A X-ray image of the breast produced by mammography.

Mandible Jawbone.

Marionette Lines The vertical creases that form in the corners of the mouth towards the jowls.

Mastopexy Breast lift procedure that re-shapes the breast with or without nipple repositioning.

Melanin The pigment that gives skin its color.

Melanoma The deadliest form of skin cancer characterized by a black or dark brown pigmented tumor.

Mentoplasty Plastic surgery of the chin whereby its shape or size is altered.

Micro-dermabrasion 'Micro-dermabrasion' or 'derma-peeling' or 'micro-abrasion' is a mechanical blasting of the face with sterile microparticles that abrade or rub off the very top skin layer, then vacuuming out the particles and the dead skin.

Microabrasion A tooth-whitening procedure using an abrasive combined with a hydrochloric acid.

Mid-face-lift Also referred to as a "cheek lift," a surgical procedure designed to lift sagging areas in the mid-face, including around the cheekbone areas below the eyes.

Midline An imaginary vertical line that divides the face or body into two equal areas.

Milia Tiny skin cysts that resemble whiteheads.

Mitral valve prolapse Cardiopathy resulting from the mitral valve not regulating the flow of blood between the left atrium and left ventricle of the heart.

Mohs Surgery The destruction of malignant, infected, or gangrenous tissue by the application of chemicals. The technique is used successfully to remove skin cancers. A procedure that removes superficial cancers using fixation with a caustic or corrosive substance, such as zinc chloride.

Monitored Anesthesia Care Also called 'local with intravenous sedation' and 'twilight', where medications are given intravenously to induce a state of sleepiness and relieve pain, supplemented with local anesthetic injections. Your surgeon can talk to you and you will be able to answer him, although won't remember anything when you wake up.

Musculature The system or arrangement of muscles in a body or a body part.

Myasthenia Abnormal muscular weakness or fatigue.

N

Nasal Labial Folds The region of the face between the nose and the corners of the lip, commonly referred to as 'smile lines'.

Nasion The depression at the root of the nose that indicates the junction where the forehead ends and the bridge of the nose begins.

Necrosis Dead skin cells.

Non ablative laser resurfacing A new class of lasers that does not produce a deep burn and provides a much less invasive treatment.

Non-comedogenic Products that are formulated not to clog the pores and cause pimples.

O

Onlay Porcelain filling that protects a tooth by covering the chewing surface, can also be made from metals.

Orbicularis Oculi The muscular body of the eyelid encircling the eye and comprising the palpebral, orbital, and lacrimal muscles. It arises from the nasal part of the frontal bone, the frontal process of the maxilla in front of the lacrimal groove, and the anterior surface of the medial palpebral ligament. The palpebral muscle functions to close the eyelid gently; the orbital muscle functions to close it more energetically, such as in winking.

Orbit The cavity in the skull where the eyeballs, eye muscles, nerves and blood vessels rest.

Orthodontia the branch of dentistry dealing with the prevention or correction of irregularities of the teeth.

Orthodontist a dentist specializing in the prevention or correction of irregularities of the teeth.

Osseointegration The growth action of bone tissue as it assimilates surgically implanted devices or prostheses to be used as either replacement parts or as anchors.

Osteotomy The operation of dividing a bone or of cutting a piece out of it.

Otoplasty Reparative or plastic surgery of the auricle of the ear.

Outpatient Surgery Ambulatory surgery in which you are discharged later the same day from the recovery room in a hospital, office surgical suite, or clinic.

P

PABA Para-aminobenzoic acid. Found in the vitamin B complex. Used as an ingredient in some sunscreen products.

Pectoralis The muscle that is located between the rib cage and the chest tissue.

Petrolatum Used in creams, it softens and soothes skin. Forms a film to prevent moisture loss.

pH The degree of acidity or alkalinity in the solution of products.

Periareolar The area around the areola.

Periodontal disease A disease that attacks the gum and bone and around the teeth.

Phenol Peeling formula applied to the skin to lighten pigment, soften wrinkles and improve scars, considered to be a deep and more invasive peel.

Phlebitis Inflammation of a vein.

Photoaging Damage to the skin due to cumulative exposure to the sun; i.e. wrinkles, age spots, fine lines.

Photosensitivity Chemicals or topical ingredients that cause the skin to be reactive when exposed to sunlight such as inflammation, hyperpigmentation and swelling.

Plaque A sticky film containing bacteria that forms on the teeth.

Platysma A thin sheet of muscle located just beneath the skin of the chin and neck.

Platysmal Bands Vertical strands of the muscle of the neck that can become more prominent with age and are often sutured or tightened during a face or necklift.

Polysaccharide Any of a class of carbohydrates, such as starch and cellulose, consisting of a number of monosaccharides joined by glycosidic bonds.

Porcelain Veneers A thin layer of porcelain adhered to a surface of a tooth to repair or change the color and/or shape.

Pore Small opening of the sweat glands of the skin.

Post A metal or ceramic reinforcement inserted into a tooth that has undergone a root canal procedure to straighten it.

Procerus Muscle that works with the corrugator muscles and contributes to the vertical frown lines between the eyebrows.

Psoriasis A noncontagious inflammatory skin disease characterized by recurring reddish patches covered with silvery scales.

PT/PTT A blood test to determine the blood coagulation factor.

Ptosis Pronounced (toe-sis), a term for drooping as in eyelids, breasts and brows.

R

Rectus Any of various straight muscles, such as, the abdomen, eye, neck, and thigh.

Resorcinol In mild solutions, used as an antiseptic and as a soothing preparation for itchy skin.

Retin-A (Tretinoin) A topical medication derived from Vitamin A that is used to treat photoaging and acne.

Retinol A gentler non-prescription strength alternative to Retinoic Acid. Retinol is a fact, active form of Vitamin A that works deep under the surface of the skin to visibly reduce lines and wrinkles.

Rhytidectomy (Face-lift) Surgical procedure which rejuvenates the face by tightening the underlying musculature, removing excess fat deposits, and redraping sagging skin of the lower face and neck. Incisions are placed in the hairline and around the ears and/or under the chin.

Root The part of the tooth that is usually anchored into the jawbone.

Rosacea A common skin condition of the face, nose, cheeks, forehead that results in redness, pimples, dilated blood vessels and occasional pustules.

S

Saline Salt water commonly used as a filler for breast implants and in the course of administering intravenous fluids.

Schirmer's Test A test that assesses tear production in the eyes and is helpful in treating dry eye syndrome.

Scleral Show Lower eyelid retraction, which exposes the sclera (white part of the eyeball), below the pupil.

Sclerotherapy The injection of one of several solutions through a small needle directly into a vein to cause it to collapse.

Sepsis A reaction of the body to bacteria that circulate in the blood, characterized by chills and fever.

Septoplasty An operation to unblock clogged sinuses in order to improve breathing.

Septum The separating wall in the nose between the left and right nasal passages.

Seroma A collection of clear fluid that may occur under the skin following surgery.

Silastic Sheeting Patches or strips of silicone that may be applied to the skin for extended time periods to soften and reduce scarring.

Silastic A sac made of rubber and silicone, often filled with silicone or salt solution.

Silicone A synthetic substance used in a gel-like form in silicone breast implants, in a liquid injectable form for facial areas, and in other medical devices.

Sinus X-rays An image of the sinus cavities.

SMA 12 A Sequential Multiple Analyzer 12 is used to perform several different blood tests.

SMAS The superficial musculoaponeurotic system (SMAS), is a layer of tissue that covers the deeper structures in the cheek area and touches the superficial muscle covering the lower face and neck called the platysma. The SMAS is often lifted and repositioned during the facelift procedure.

SPF (Sun Protection Factor) A scale used to rate the level of protection sunscreens provide from UVB rays of the sun.

Spider Veins (Telangiectasias) Dilated or broken blood vessels near the surface of the skin.

Spinal blocks A form of anesthesia that numbs the lower two-thirds of the body.

Steroids Any of a large number of hormonal substances with similar basic chemical structure, produced mainly in the adrenal cortex and gonads.

Stratum Corneum Surface layer of epidermis.

Striae Commonly known as stretchmarks, cause by thinning of the underlying skin layer (dermis) that appear first as red, raised lines, then darken and flatten gradually to form shiny whitened streaks.

Subglandular Under the gland, typically of the breast

Submental Referring to the area below the chin

Subpectoral Also called submuscular, referring to the area below the pectoralis muscle where a breast implant may be placed

Subperiosteal A term for a procedure that goes deep into multiple layers; a lift in which all tissues are separated from the underlying bone structure, thereby considered more invasive, as in brow, face, etc.

Suction Assisted Lipectomy (Liposuction) A procedure in which localized collections of fat are removed from the face and/or body by using a high vacuum device through small incisions.

Sunblock A physical sunscreen or a barrier against the sun's ultraviolet rays. Available in creams or ointments.

T

Tartar Cement-like substance that forms when plaque is not effectively removed from the teeth.

Tartaric Acid A type of glycolic acid derived from apples.

Tazarotene A prescription topical retinoid (vitamin A derivative) approved for treating mild to moderate plaque psoriasis.

Tempromandibular Joint (TMJ) The joint that connects the upper and lower jaws.

Thrombosis The obstruction of a blood vessel by a clot formed at the site of obstruction.

Thyroid The endocrine gland, located in front of the neck, which regulates body metabolism. It secretes a hormone known as thyroxin.

Tiplasty A nose augmentation.

Tissue Engineering The science of production of human tissue ex vivo, (outside of the human body) as in growing cartilage in tissue culture.

Tissue Glue A compound used instead of stitches or staples in surgery.

Titanium Dioxide A non-chemical, common agent used in sunscreen products that works by physically blocking the sun. It may be used alone or in combination with other agents.

Tocopherol Chemical name for vitamin E, an antioxidant

Tram Flap Acronym for 'transverse rectus abdominis myuocutaneous', a breast reconstruction method whereby a flap of abdominal fat and skin is moved to the chest wall to form a newly reconstructed breast.

Tragus A small extension of the auricular cartilage of the ear, anterior to the external meatus.

Transaxillary An incision placed under the arm for access during surgery, as in breast augmentation.

Transumbilical An approach whereby the incision is placed in the umbilicus (belly button) through which breast implants may be moved into position.

Tretinoin A derivative of vitamin A.

Trichloroacetic acid A colorless, deliquescent, corrosive, crystalline compound, used topically as an astringent and antiseptic.

Tumescent A method of anesthesia where large volumes of local anesthetic and saline solution are injected to swell the area to be operated on, commonly used in liposuction and body contouring procedures.

Twilight Anesthesia See monitored anesthesia care.

U

Ultrasound Application of a sound wave, a mechanical vibration of more than 16,000 cycles per second.

Umbilicus Belly button or navel.

Undermining Surgical separation of tissues from their underlying structures.

Urethra The canal through which urine is discharged from the bladder in most mammals and through which semen is discharged in the male.

UVA Long wavelengths emitted by the sun which take longer to produce a burn than UVB but penetrate deeper into the skin to cause sun damage.

UVB Short wavelengths emitted by the sun, which are known to cause premature aging and skin cancer.

V

Varicose Veins Enlarged, swollen and dilated veins just below the surface of the skin, commonly found in the legs and caused by the valves becoming filled with blood

Vector The direction of pull, as in face-lifting, etc.

Vermillion Border The external pinkish-to-red area of the upper and lower lips. It extends from the junction of the lips with surrounding facial skin on the exterior to the labial mucosa within the mouth.

W

Wavelength The distance between a given point on one wave cycle and the corresponding point on the next successive wave cycle, the light of the wavelength produces a pure color.

Witch's Chin Pointy or droopy chin syndrome.

X

Xanthoma A fatty deposit in the skin that may appear on the lower eyelids or elsewhere.

Y

YAG Abbreviation for yttrium aluminum garnet, a crystal used in some types of lasers.

Z

Zinc Oxide Chemical ingredient that has soothing and astringent qualities that can block ultraviolet rays of the sun.

Z-plasty A z-shaped incisional technique used to conceal a scar in the natural skin creases.

Zygomatic Arch An arch formed by the temporal process of the zygomatic bone with the zygomatic process of the temporal bone. The tendon of the temporal muscle passes beneath it.

Subject Index

T

User Guide

The CD in the back of this book is a searchable registry of cosmetic doctors and dentists. You can use this registry to search for qualified cosmetic doctors and dentists in your area or across the nation.

1. Insert the CD into your CD drive. The application may open automatically. If not, open the CD and double-click on **start.htm**.

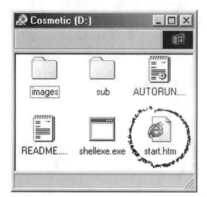
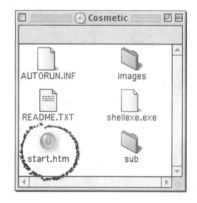

Windows   Macintosh

2. The application will give you the option to choose either "to Register" or "to Launch Application". If it's your first time using this CD, please choose "to Register".

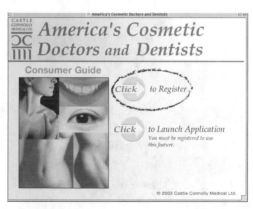

3. In the Registration window you will first be asked to fill out a short form. You will find the 12-digit serial number requested on this form inside the CD envelope (behind the CD). Please fill out the form completely, and click **Register Now**.

4. A second registration form will appear requesting additional information. The corresponding fields from the previous screen will already be filled. To complete the registration process, supply the additional information. *Only the items in red are required.* Once you click **Register Now**, your password will be sent to the email address you have provided. *Please ensure that you provide a current email address.*

5. Once you have received the password, return to the CD application window, enter your email address and password and click Launch Application.

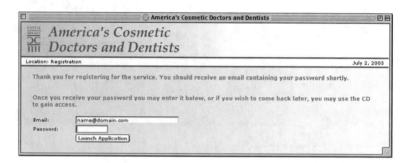

Or if applicable place the CD in the drive and after following Step 1, click "to Launch Application").

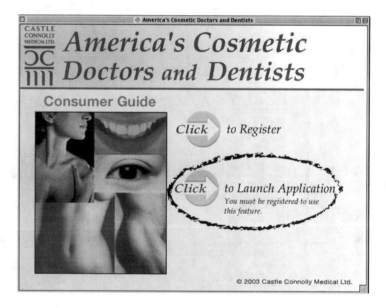

CASTLE CONNOLLY ORDER FORM

I want to order the following Castle Connolly Guides
at these discounted prices (15%):

America's Top Doctors, 3rd edition   # ___ of books at $25.46 $_____

Top Doctors:
     New York Metro Area, 7th edition   # ___ of books at $21.21 $_____
     Chicago Metro Area, 3nd edition   # ___ of books at $21.21 $_____

How to Find the Best Doctors:
     Florida   # ___ of books at $21.21 $_____

America's Cosmetic Doctors
and Dentists   # ___ of books at $25.46 $_____

The Buyer's Guide to Choosing
the Best Healthcare   # ___ of books at $11.01 $_____

The ABCs of HMOs: How To
Get The Best From Managed Care   # ___ of books at $10.16 $_____

                                     Subtotal $_____

      *NY residents, please add 8.25% sales tax $_____
       **NJ residents, please add 6% sales tax $_____

Add $4.99 per book for shipping and handling: # ___ of books x $4.99 $_____

                                     TOTAL $_____

Please fill in the following information (please print):

Name: _____

Address: _____

City: _____

State: _____ Zip: _____

Phone (day): _____ (eve): _____

E-mail: _____

___ Check or Money Order enclosed
      (payable to Castle Connolly Medical Ltd.)
___ Credit Card: please circle one   Amex   MC   Visa

Card #: _____

Exp. Date: _____ Today's Date: _____

Signature: _____

Mail to: Castle Connolly Medical Ltd. 42 West 24th Street, New York, NY 10010
or fax to: (212) 367-0964
Order online: www.castleconnolly.com

About the Authors

Wendy Lewis has been an insider to the field of aesthetic medicine for two decades. She holds a BA from Columbia University - Barnard College and did her post graduate work at Fordham University Graduate School of Business Administration. Lewis began her career as a Practice Administrator for two prominent New York aesthetic plastic surgeons, and became an internationally reknown cosmetic surgery and skin care consultant who fills a void between medical liaison and beauty advisor. She has been called a "KNIFE COACH" who helps clients, both women and men, with all their image concerns. Lewis sees clients face to face in New York and London, or via phone from all over the world. She is the author of seven books, including *The Beauty Batttle* (Laurel Glen), is the Editor of her own beauty journal, *WL Beauty Watch*, and has had more than 200 articles published in magazines, newspapers and journals on two continents. Lewis is in demand as a guest speaker and has been seen on Today New York, CNN, Good Morning America, the *New York Times Style Section*, *New York Magazine*, *Vogue*, *Tatler*, *Harpers & Queen*, and many others. 1-877-WLBEAUTY, wlbeauty@aol.com, www.wlbeauty.com

John J. Connolly, Ed.D., is the president and CEO of Castle Connolly Medical Ltd, publishers of the Top Doctors since 1991. For more information see About the Publishers on page ix.

chapter 8

Acknowledgments

The publishers would like to thank the entire staff for their many hours and days of intense and precise work on this guide in order to further its goal of assisting consumers in making the best healthcare choices.

We offer a special thank you to those physicians and dentists who offered their constructive comments and support, and to the medical and dental professional organizations for their assistance in creating this guide.

In particular, we would like to thank:

Anne Akers, *Special Advisor*

AE Freisler, *Research Project Manager* and her research team

Peter Cusack, *Designer*

Vicky Klukkert, *Editorial Associate*

Anne Pradoura, *Public Relations Associate*

Castle Connolly Executive Management:

President & CEO: John J. Connolly, Ed.D

Vice President, Research: Jean Morgan, MD

Vice President, Business Development: William Liss-Levinson, Ph.D.

Director, Information Technology: Michael Pitkin

CUSTOMER FEEDBACK OFFER

We would appreciate your help improving our guide. If you will take a few minutes to complete this survey, we will give you a *free copy* of a Healthcare Choice Guide.

How did you find out about this book?

☐ From a Friend   ☐ TV   ☐ Newspaper   ☐ Radio

☐ From a Doctor   ☐ Bookstore   ☐ Other _____

Why did you purchase this book?

☐ Needed a Specialist   ☐ As a General Reference Guide

☐ Needed a Primary Care Physician   ☐ Other _____

Did you use this book to find any physicians?

☐ No   ☐ Yes – If yes, ☐ 1 doctor   ☐ 2-3 doctors   ☐ 4 or more doctors

Where do you primarily use this book?

☐ Home   ☐ Office

Did you use this book as a reference to find a doctor for a friend or relative?

☐ No   ☐ Yes – If yes, # of times _____

Did you loan this book to a friend or relative?

☐ No   ☐ Yes – If yes, # of times _____

Do you have any suggestions for improving the book? _____

_____

_____

Are there any other books you would like to see us publish? _____

_____

_____

To Thank You for Helping Us...

Please check the ONE Healthcare Choice Guide that you wish to receive:

☐ *Board and Care Facilities and Adult Foster Homes*

☐ *Catching Costly Billing Errors*

☐ *Choosing a Chiropractor*

☐ *Choosing a Comprehensive Women's Health Center*

☐ *Choosing a Dentist*

☐ *Choosing a Diagnostic Cardiology Center*

☐ *Choosing a Diagnostic Imaging Center*

☐ *Choosing a Hospital*

☐ *Choosing a Nursing Home*

☐ *Choosing a Primary Care Doctor*

☐ *Choosing a Specialist*

☐ *Choosing a Veterinarian*

☐ *Choosing an Ambulatory Surgery Center*

☐ *Choosing an Assisted Living Facility*

☐ *Choosing Eldercare Advisors*

☐ *Family Caregivers*

☐ *Home Healthcare*

☐ *Home Modification for Elder-Friendly Living*

☐ *Rehabilitation Services*

☐ *Understanding Health Plans*

Name: _____

Address: _____

City: _____ State: _____ Zip Code _____

Mail or fax to:

Castle Connolly Medical Ltd. 42 West 24th Street, New York, NY 10010

Fax: (212) 367-0964 www.castleconnolly.com

DOCTOR-PATIENT ADVISOR

Doctor-Patient Advisor is a Castle Connolly Medical Ltd., service providing one on one consultations with a Healthcare Advocate to individuals who have extremely serious or complex medical problems or to anyone who feels he/she needs assistance finding the right physician for any purpose. Each client will receive personalized assistance from these physician-supervised nurses in identifying the appropriate top specialists for his/her condition. The Healthcare Advocate will utilize the extensive Castle Connolly Medical Ltd. database of physicians and hospitals to locate and facilitate access to the best resources to meet the client's needs. Fee: $695.00. For further information call (212) 367-8400 x 16.

For further information on physicians and hospitals please visit the Castle Connolly Web site at
www.CastleConnolly.com or at
www.AmericasCosmeticDoctors.com

LICENSE AGREEMENT:

The purchaser is hereby licensed to use the Software, from the date of purchase until November 1, 2004, to access Castle Connolly Medical Ltd.'s proprietary, internet-based database of plastic surgeons, dermatologists, and related medical providers. This License is not transferable. The Software may be used only by the purchaser and his or her immediate family, only in the purchaser's home and/or office, and shall not be copied, transmitted, decompiled or reverse engineered. Any use inconsistent with the foregoing shall be grounds for immediate termination of this License Agreement, in addition to all other remedies available to Castle Connolly Medical Ltd. at law and in equity.